The Melanoma Book

The Melanoma Book

A Complete Guide to Prevention and Treatment

Howard L. Kaufman, M.D.

A Lark Production

GOTHAM BOO

616.99
KAUFMAN

GOTHAM BOOKS
Published by Penguin Group (USA) Inc.
375 Hudson Street, New York, New York 10014, U.S.A.
Penguin Group (Canada), 10 Alcorn Avenue, Toronto, Ontario, Canada M4V 3B2 (a division
of Pearson Penguin Canada Inc.); Penguin Books Ltd, 80 Strand, London WC2R 0RL, England; Penguin Ireland, 25 St Stephen's Green, Dublin 2, Ireland (a division of Penguin Books
Ltd); Penguin Group (Australia), 250 Camberwell Road, Camberwell, Victoria 3124, Australia
(a division of Pearson Australia Group Pty Ltd); Penguin Books India Pvt Ltd, 11 Community
Centre, Panchsheel Park, New Delhi - 110 017, India; Penguin Group (NZ), Cnr Airborne
and Rosedale Roads, Albany, Auckland, New Zealand (a division of Pearson New Zealand Ltd);
Penguin Books (South Africa) (Pty) Ltd, 24 Sturdee Avenue, Rosebank, Johannesburg 2196,
South Africa

Penguin Books Ltd, Registered Offices: 80 Strand, London WC2R 0RL, England

Published by Gotham Books, a division of Penguin Group (USA) Inc.

First printing, May 2005
10 9 8 7 6 5 4 3 2 1

Library of Congress Cataloging-in-Publication Data
Kaufman, Howard L.
    The melanoma book : a complete guide to prevention and treatment, including the early de-
tection self-exam body map / by Howard L. Kaufman.
    p. cm.
Includes bibliographical references and index.
ISBN 1-59240-126-0 (alk. paper)
    1. Melanoma—Popular works. I. Title.
RC280.M37K38 2005
616.99'477—dc22   2004060794

Printed in the United States of America
Set in Janson Text
Designed by Rachel Reiss

PUBLISHER'S NOTE
Neither the publisher nor the author is engaged in rendering professional advice or services to
the individual reader. The ideas, procedures, and suggestions contained in this book are not in-
tended as a substitute for consulting with your physician. All matters regarding your health require medical supervision. Neither the author nor the publisher shall be liable or responsible
for any loss or damage allegedly arising from any information or suggestion in this book.

This book is dedicated to my patients, who continue to teach me to be a better physician, and to Gail DeRaffele, R.N., whose dedication to providing compassionate and expert care for our patients is a constant source of inspiration.

Contents

Foreword

GIVEN THE RAPID pace of changes in cancer medicine, it is not surprising that cancer specialists often fall behind in conveying their knowledge to patients and their families. This is particularly true for malignant melanoma, a disease too often missed or mistreated in its early, potentially curable stages. I was delighted to read this clear and comprehensive book written by Dr. Howard Kaufman, a respected surgical oncologist and melanoma specialist at Columbia University.

As you might expect, the book is divided into chapters covering prevention, diagnosis, staging, and treatment. What is unexpected—and highly successful—is the way Dr. Kaufman seamlessly combines scientific information and practical tips. He includes all the medical terminology in the text, as well as in a separate glossary, and each term is carefully defined. If you or someone you love has been diagnosed with melanoma, you know that such demystification of medical jargon is invaluable.

Throughout the book, Dr. Kaufman favors short tables to summarize important points and avoids color pictures that might be more anxiety-provoking than helpful. At the end of each chapter, he includes a case study and a list of questions for patients to ask their doctors. Although each chapter might stand alone as a useful overview, all are linked by several critically important tenets. Among these is the concept of multidisciplinary treatment; an essential section explains the "doctors who deal with melanoma" and reminds us that no one doctor handles all aspects of melanoma. Another vital point is the importance of early detection and adequate treatment—and the fact that biopsy is not treatment.

More subtle, but clear, is the emphasis on long-term management and a multidisciplinary treatment plan, not to be confused with one-time treatment of acute disease. As a surgical oncologist who has been treating melanoma patients for forty years, I know that the combination of surgical and non-surgical interventions can control melanoma and preserve quality of life for many years.

I also know that the best caregivers deliver knowledge as well as treatment. What does "AJCC stage" mean? When is a PET scan necessary? What should you do if your sentinel node is positive? These questions deserve careful responses. *The Melanoma Book* responds with a scope and consistency that will help you maintain a proactive approach to melanoma. On behalf of melanoma specialists everywhere, I thank Dr. Kaufman for giving patients and professionals this valuable resource.

Donald L. Morton, M.D., F.A.C.S.
Medical Director and Surgeon-in-Chief
John Wayne Cancer Institute
Santa Monica, California

The Melanoma Book

Introduction

WHO IS LIVING with melanoma?

A forty-six-year-old man whose barber noticed a small black mole on his scalp during a regular haircut. An otherwise healthy eight-year-old girl, who came home from school one afternoon complaining of blurred vision. A thirty-two-year-old woman who had been suffering from garden-variety hemorrhoids for several months.

These three patients represent how cunning and varied a melanoma diagnosis can be. The locations it can emerge on the body and its lack of symptoms make it a challenging disease indeed to find and treat, as I know only too well. I've treated hundreds of patients for melanoma in the last fourteen years. In the years to come, I expect to see thousands more because *the number of new melanoma patients worldwide is rising at a rate faster than that of any other cancer*. Striking every age, gender, and socioeconomic group, melanoma is quickly becoming one of the most familiar cancers among the general population. Already *melanoma has become the most common cancer among women aged twenty-five to twenty-nine*. Among women aged thirty to thirty-four, it is second only to lung cancer (the leading cancer in both men and women).

That's why I decided to write this book. With such a dramatic rise in the incidence of melanoma, I felt it was more important than ever before to provide the many patients and families beyond the scope of my practice with a basic understanding of malignant melanoma, what it is, how it is diagnosed and treated, and where to go for appropriate care. As both a practicing physician and a clinical investigator, I'm in the unique position of being directly involved with cutting-edge treatment for this deadly disease. With early detection melanoma has a high rate of cure, but there is a great deal of controversy surrounding the treatment of the disease in its later stages. Despite a significant amount of research, the survival rate for patients with metastatic melanoma continues to be only 10–15 percent. And there is no consensus among experts as to the best course of action. Patients and their families faced with a melanoma diagnosis are understandably confused and afraid.

Given that melanoma often strikes previously healthy individuals in the prime of their lives, many find themselves ill prepared and poorly equipped for the medical and psychological journey on which they are forced to embark. Confronted with a melanoma diagnosis, a patient may be overwhelmed with questions:

- What is malignant melanoma?
- How is this disease different from other types of skin cancer?
- Why did I get this?
- What kind of doctor should I consult for this condition?
- How should I be treated?
- Can my disease be prevented or cured?

I hope to answer these questions and more in the following pages.

The proper care of malignant melanoma requires the cooperation of many different types of doctors with expertise in a wide variety of areas, including dermatology, surgery, oncology, radiation oncology, diagnostic radiology, and pathology. There are effective treatments for malignant melanoma when it is found at an early stage. It is essential to learn about malignant melanoma, because the more you know about it, the greater the chances of early detection. Then you can develop a logical treatment plan with experts in the management of this disease.

At the Melanoma Center of Columbia University Medical Center, we have established a multidisciplinary team approach to the diagnosis and treatment of malignant melanoma. This has been instrumental in providing the latest diagnostic techniques, surgical procedures, new treatments, and proper follow-up care for patients with malignant melanoma. Recent discoveries in molecular biology, genetics, and immunology are revolutionizing our approach to the malignant melanoma patient. By bringing together basic scientists, clinical practitioners, nursing specialists, and public-health experts, we are providing the most comprehensive care for our patients. Changes in biomedical research and clinical sciences are happening at a rapid pace, and it will be increasingly important for patients and physicians to obtain the most up-to-date information when making medical decisions.

I have based this book on the collective wisdom and work of the Columbia University Medical Center team. While I don't insist that our approach is applicable for all patients, my hope is that the information provided and the insight into our procedures and decision-making processes will help patients and their families understand what is happening and why. I offer you the same state-of-the-art research findings and treatment options from which my patients benefit at Columbia. No matter where you live, if melanoma strikes, you can use this book to understand the disease and begin the process of healing.

The book is divided into four main parts: prevention, diagnosis, treatment, and research. Part One explains melanoma and how it differs from other types of skin cancer. It also discusses the causes of melanoma and explains how melanoma may be prevented. In Part Two, I lead you step-by-step through the specific ways we diagnose and categorize, or *stage*, melanoma. Part Three is all about treating melanoma, from basic biopsy to experimental laser surgery, adjuvant therapy, and chemotherapy. No doubt many of you will want to turn directly to that section. I conclude with Part Four, which covers the most current research, including cytokine, vaccine, and genetic therapies as well as a thorough discussion of clinical trials.

My goal with this book is to help you organize key issues, understand the options, and make informed decisions about diagnostic and treatment procedures. Even when the disease is advanced, there are often dramatic responses, and occasionally even cures. By better understanding

melanoma, you will learn how to live with the disease, and perhaps prevent it from occurring in your loved ones.

I hope that with the help of the information in this book, you and
your loved ones never face a diagnosis of melanoma. But, if you do, here
is all the information you need to cope with the diagnosis and increase
the chances of survival.

PART ONE

Preventing Melanoma

CHAPTER ONE

What Is Melanoma?

THE MOMENT YOU or a loved one has been diagnosed with melanoma, questions begin to crowd out almost all other thoughts: *What does melanoma mean? What's the difference between it and other skin cancers? What are the implications for me and my family?* Before you can begin to grasp the diagnosis and start the recovery process, you need clear answers.

The good news is that most melanomas are found early, and the cure rate is approximately 85 percent in these cases. Even when melanoma is found in the advanced stages, treatments can often be remarkably successful.

Simply stated, melanoma is a type of skin cancer that arises from the melanocytes, one particular type of skin cell. Melanoma occurs when the melanocytes become severely abnormal, start dividing uncontrollably, and eventually spread to other parts of the body, sometimes resulting in death.

Most of our cells grow and divide continually. This process is essential for replacing old and worn-out cells, such as on the surface of the skin. The critical balance of cell growth, division, and death is tightly regulated by the genes, which are made up of a substance called DNA. When the DNA is altered, the normal life cycle of cells becomes impaired or out of control. Uncontrolled division of cells results in the growth of a tumor ("tumor" comes from the Latin word for "mass").

Many things can cause alterations or mutations in DNA, including hereditary factors, exposure to radiation and ultraviolet light, certain toxic chemicals (such as tobacco), and certain viruses. Whatever the cause of the mutations, if the cells continue to divide without stopping, a growth or mass will form: cancer. When this process occurs in the skin, it is called skin cancer.

The severity of the disease is also determined by the ability of the cells to grow into a large size and then spread to other parts of the body, a process called *metastasis*. Cancers that are more aggressive in their growth and can spread to other parts of the body are called *malignant*. Cancers that remain small in size and do not spread are called *benign*, and generally behave in a less threatening manner. *This is true not just for skin cancers, but for all cancers in the body.*

The names of different forms of cancer are based on their classification as benign or malignant. Benign cancers usually end with the suffix "-oma," such as *lipoma*, which refers to a benign growth of fat cells that occurs just under the skin. In contrast, malignant cancers are often called "carcinomas," such as *breast carcinoma* or *colon carcinoma*. Melanoma is one of the few exceptions to this rule, reflecting the early misconception that melanomas were benign cancers with little tendency to spread. When it became clear that melanomas could grow to large sizes and could spread to almost any other organ in the body, the medical term was changed to *malignant melanoma* in order to denote the more serious nature of this type of cancer.

Although this book focuses on malignant melanoma, many other kinds of skin cancer exist. These other skin cancers are much more common and usually are easier to cure than melanoma. The type of skin cancer and its severity depends on which cell is the source of the cancer. So in order to understand melanoma and other skin cancers, it's helpful to put them in the context of the normal structures and cells of the skin.

The Structure of the Skin

While its primary function is to protect the body from invading germs, chemicals, water, temperature, and other conditions or irritating substances, the skin also performs other vital functions including:

- regulating body temperature
- fighting infections in conjunction with the body's immune system
- protecting us from ultraviolet damage by the sun
- regulating Vitamin D metabolism

The skin is a complex body organ comprised of two major layers: the epidermis and the dermis. Each of these two main layers contains highly specialized skin cells arranged in sub-layers.

The Epidermis

The epidermis, the layer closest to the skin's surface, contains five sub-layers, or *strata*. The outermost sub-layers provide a critical protective barrier for the body (see Table 1-1). Generally considered "dead" because their cells do not divide, these outermost layers continually slough off. Cells in the deepest sub-layer (the *stratum basale*) divide and replace the cells in the outer layers, completely renewing the skin every twenty-five to fifty days.

Melanocytes are specialized cells that produce melanin, the dark brown pigment responsible for darkening the skin. Melanocytes are located in the deepest epidermal sub-layer (the *stratum basale*). In response to direct sunlight, these cells produce melanin, which causes the skin to become darker and is visible to the human eye as tanning. Melanin also helps protect against ultraviolet radiation and sun damage.

The activity of the melanocytes determines the natural color of the skin. In other words, your skin color depends not on the number of melanocytes present, but on how much melanin they make.

Table 1-1. The five layers of the epidermis and their function

Layer of the Epidermis	Function
Stratum corneum	Outermost layer; protects the body from external forces
Stratum lucidum	Provides cells and keratin for the outer layers of skin
Stratum granulosum	Produces proteins that cement the skin and helps protect the body from water and other outside forces
Stratum spinosum	Provides a layer of strong attachments that prevents abrasions of the skin
Stratum basale	Innermost layer of epidermis, where melanocytes are located; provides a source for cells in the outer layers of epidermis

The Dermis

The dermis is the larger, inner layer of the skin and, like the epidermis, contains sub-layers (see Table 1-2). To better understand melanoma, it is important to know that the deeper (*reticular*) layer contains blood vessels, lymphatic vessels, and larger nerves of the skin. The vessels in this layer can pick up specialized cells—*including melanoma cells*—and carry them to the lymph nodes. From there, melanomas may travel through the lymphatic and vascular systems and cause cancers in almost any other part of the body.

Table 1-2. The two layers of the dermis and their function

Layer of the Dermis	Function
Papillary dermis: *thin layer*	Contains papilla that hold the epidermis and dermis together

Layer of the Dermis	Function
Reticular dermis: *thick layer*	Contains blood vessels involved in regulation of temperature
	Contains sweat glands for temperature control and pheromone release
	Contains nerve endings and specialized cells that regulate the sense of touch
	Contains hair follicles and sebaceous glands

Cancers of the Skin

When I examine a new patient with a skin growth, also known as a lesion, the first question I always ask is whether it has changed from its usual size or shape. This is a crucial question, because nearly all cancerous lesions will exhibit a change. In fact, such changes are the most common reason why people seek medical attention for a skin growth. If a lesion has been present since childhood and has not changed in any way, the likelihood of a serious cancer is much lower.

The second question I ask is whether the skin lesion is pigmented. Whether or not I see pigment is key because melanin is a clue that the melanocyte is the source of the growth, which raises concern about melanoma. Please note that *not all melanoma lesions will have pigment.* About five percent of melanomas have no pigment at all and are called **amelanotic melanomas**. Nonetheless, the first distinction that your dermatologist or pathologist will make is whether the skin growth is pigmented or non-pigmented.

Cancer can develop from almost any cell in the skin (or elsewhere in the body), but certain cells are far more frequent culprits than others. Non-pigmented cells—as opposed to pigmented melanocytes—are the predominant source of skin cancers.

Non-Pigmented Skin Cancer

The two most common non-pigmented skin cancers are basal cell carcinoma and squamous cell carcinoma, named after the respective cells that cause them. Fortunately, the most common variety of non-pigmented skin cancer is relatively easy to cure (see Table 1-3).

Basal cell carcinoma, the most common human cancer, likely accounts for about one quarter of all cancers in the United States. Parts of the body that are exposed to the sun, such as the face—especially the nose and scalp—are the most frequent sites of basal cell carcinoma. Most experienced dermatologists will be able to recognize a basal cell carcinoma, although some are trickier to identify. One type that happens to produce pigment, for example, can be confused with a melanoma.

Although fairly common, basal cell carcinoma only spreads (metastasizes) to other parts of the body in fewer than 0.1 percent of cases. But treatment is still required since it can disrupt the surrounding normal tissues. Basal cell carcinomas on the nose, ear, and eyelid are often more prone to recurrence, so it is important to make sure that they are completely removed or treated.

Patients with basal cell carcinoma should be examined at least once a year by a dermatologist. If basal cell carcinomas recur, they usually do so within one to five years but may develop at any time. In addition, patients with one basal cell carcinoma may develop other basal cell carcinomas.

Squamous cell carcinoma occurs when the keratin-producing cells in the skin divide without control. Squamous cell carcinoma is the second most common skin cancer, occurring in about 100,000 people each year in the United States. Those who have difficulty tanning and tend to burn when exposed to the sun for a prolonged period of time appear to be at higher risk for developing squamous cell carcinomas. People with fair complexions and those of Celtic descent also have a higher frequency.

Like basal cell carcinomas, this cancer also occurs most commonly on sun-exposed parts of the body and is slightly more common in men than women. But squamous cell carcinoma is much more serious because it is more aggressive and grows more rapidly, causing local destruction of normal tissues, and it has the potential for metastasizing to other parts of the body.

Squamous cell carcinomas appear on the skin as slightly raised and reddish areas and may grow over a period of several weeks to months. Squamous cell carcinomas that occur on the lips and ear are usually more difficult to control than those occurring elsewhere. The severity of squamous cell carcinomas depends on their size, how deep they are located within the layers of the skin, and on the characteristics of the cells involved. This information can only be obtained by a biopsy and examination under a microscope. Some forms of squamous cell carcinoma are very thin and located only in the epidermis and are usually easier to control.

When squamous cell carcinomas spread, they may send cells to the lymph nodes nearby or to internal organs. Always have the lymph node areas of the body examined if you have a squamous cell carcinoma. In cases where the cancer is very large or the cells are very aggressive, further evaluation of the internal organs may be necessary by obtaining a special X-ray known as a CT or CAT scan.

Since squamous cell carcinoma can recur and because a second squamous cell carcinoma can develop, it is important to see a dermatologist on a regular basis after having a squamous cell carcinoma. A good rule of thumb is to have a full skin and lymph node evaluation every three months for the first year after treatment, then every six months during the second year, and once a year after that.

RARE FORMS OF NON-PIGMENTED SKIN CANCERS

Cancer can occur from any of a number of other specialized cells and structures within the skin. Although these cancers are extremely rare, they can be quite serious, even life threatening. The diagnosis of a rare non-pigmented skin cancer usually requires referral to specialists.

Cancer of the sweat glands is called **microcystic adnexal carcinoma.** More common in women, it usually occurs in middle age. People who received radiation treatment for acne and thyroid cancer may be prone to this type of cancer. Patients require close monitoring, since there is a high likelihood that the cancer may come back in the same location.

Cancer in the sebaceous glands is **sebaceous carcinoma.** These cancers occur more frequently in women, are most commonly located on the upper eyelid, and may be associated with exposure to previous radiation. In about 20 percent of the cases the cancer may spread to other sites. Occasionally sebaceous carcinomas have been linked to cancer in other organs, especially the colon and urinary tracts. Because of this relationship, patients with sebaceous carcinoma are evaluated for colon cancer and urinary tract cancers.

Atypical fibroxanthoma appears as a nodule on the head and neck region in elderly adults or on the torso, arms, and legs in younger adults. The cells involved have a spindlelike appearance. This cancer has been known to metastasize and should therefore be treated by simple excision.

A specialized cell whose function may relate to the sense of touch or to the endocrine system, the Merkel cell can develop into aggressive cancers known as **Merkel cell carcinomas.** Found most often on the head in older people, these cancers have a tendency to spread to the lymph nodes and later to internal organs.

In addition to these skin cell cancers, cancers of other parts of the body such as the breast, lung, and colon, may spread to the skin. Sometimes the cancer in the skin is the first sign of the primary cancer.

Table 1-3. Types of non-pigmented skin cancer

Type of Cancer	Characteristics
Basal cell carcinoma	Most common skin cancer; rarely spreads; several methods of effective therapy
Squamous cell carcinoma	Less common but more likely to spread; usually treated by surgery or Mohs procedure

Type of Cancer	Characteristics
Microcystic adnexal carcinoma	Cancer of the sweat glands; aggressive cancer but unlikely to spread
Sebaceous gland carcinoma	Most often occur on the eyelid and can spread; treatment is surgical excision
Atypical fibroxanthoma	Spindle-shaped cancer cells that appear as nodules; can spread; treated by Mohs procedure
Merkel cell carcinoma	Rare but aggressive cancer arising from Merkel cells; may spread to lymph nodes
Metastatic carcinoma	Cancers from internal organs that spread to the skin; prognosis depends on the type of cancer

Pigmented Skin Lesions

In addition to the non-pigmented skin lesions I've mentioned above, there is another broad category: pigmented skin lesions. They include both benign and malignant forms. Benign pigmented skin lesions, which comprise the majority, are called moles. Malignant pigmented skin lesions are called melanoma. Melanocytes, the cells that produce the pigment melanin, are the most common source of both kinds of pigmented skin growths. Melanoma occurs only when the melanocytes become severely abnormal and start dividing uncontrollably.

Moles are a normal part of the skin. When melanocytes, which are distributed in the lower layers of the epidermis throughout the body, grow in clusters with surrounding normal cells, a mole occurs. The difference between a mole and melanoma is that the melanocytes stop dividing in the mole but continue to grow without stopping in a melanoma. Moles can develop anywhere on the body that is covered by skin. The typical mole appears as a small flat or slightly raised growth of pink, tan, or brown coloration. Moles are usually symmetrical, which means the border is very smooth. Some moles may be unusual and can lead to cancer.

Everybody has moles—between ten and forty is considered normal. Both children and adults may develop new moles (although the growth of new moles is less common after about forty years of age). Sometimes moles may grow and lift off the skin, but they are usually smaller than a pencil eraser. Moles may also fade or disappear completely over time.

The number and size of moles may be important factors in predicting the risk of melanoma. Interestingly, the number of moles is genetically determined, as demonstrated by the fact that identical twins have exactly the same number of moles, but non-identical twins do not. The risk of melanoma increases in people with more than fifty moles that are larger than two millimeters in diameter and in people with five or more moles larger than five millimeters in diameter.

TYPES OF MOLES

Doctors refer to a mole as a *nevus*, and multiple moles are called *nevi*. The **common nevus** is a typical mole and is sub-categorized by the pathologist depending on where the growth is located in the layers of the skin:

- a junctional nevus occurs only in cells in the epidermis

- a compound nevus contains cells in both the epidermis and dermis

- a dermal nevus is a mole in which cells are confined to the dermis. Dermal nevi may not appear pigmented since they are below the epidermis.

The **blue nevus,** a variant of the common nevus, is named for the blue color caused by the melanin-containing cells deep within the epidermis. Most common in women, it can occur in children and young adults. These nevi develop on the scalp, hands, and feet and are considered benign lesions. But treatment by simple surgical excision is usually recommended because, on rare occasions, melanoma can develop in a blue nevus.

A common nevus occasionally develops unusual features that distinguish it from all the others. These unusual moles are called **atypical** or **dysplastic nevi,** and differ from common nevi in several ways. First, atypical nevi are larger than five millimeters in diameter. In addition, these lesions may have inconsistent coloration, irregular or notched edges, and blurry borders. These lesions are sometimes smooth, but have also been described as scaly or "pebbly."

Atypical nevi are more likely than common nevi to develop into melanoma, although the exact relationship between atypical nevi and melanoma remains the subject of some speculation among experts. Any signs of a change in a mole, including an increase in the size of the mole, change in the edges, color, or new bleeding from the mole, all warrant evaluation by a medical professional. Atypical nevi are found in about 5 percent of the general population but in 30–40 percent of patients with melanoma, suggesting a strong correlation. There are many more patients with atypical nevi that do not develop melanoma, however, so other factors are likely involved as well.

A **congenital nevus** is an elevated, pigmented lesion present at birth in some babies. These lesions, which can vary in size and be quite large, have been suspected of increasing the risk of melanoma, a rare but possible occurrence in children. The risk seems to be related to the size of the congenital nevus, with those that cover more than 5 percent of the child's body, roughly equivalent to the right leg of an average two-year-old, having a significant risk. Since almost half the melanomas arising from congenital nevi occur in the first ten years of life, large congenital nevi should be removed as early as possible.

Another lesion that can be difficult to distinguish from melanoma in children is called a **Spitz nevus** (named after the pathologist who first reported it). These are usually small pinkish nodules, although they may also be pigmented. Spitz nevi are considered benign, but must be reviewed by an experienced pathologist to make certain.

COMMON BENIGN PIGMENTED SKIN LESIONS
- Common nevus
- Blue nevus
- Atypical or dysplastic nevus
- Congenital nevus
- Spitz nevus

Now that I've described the non-pigmented skin cancers and the benign pigmented skin lesions, only one category is left: malignant pigmented skin lesions, more commonly known as melanoma.

What Is Melanoma?

The appearance of melanoma is often obvious to professionals who treat the disease on a regular basis, but there are no absolute criteria that determine if a particular lesion is a melanoma. Melanomas are as diverse in appearance as people are, and therefore a challenge to identify through visual inspection alone. Any suspicious skin lesion should be considered for a biopsy, as this is the only way to know for certain if it is a melanoma. Some melanomas may start from a mole that has been present for many years, but increases in size, changes in its borders, or begins to bleed. Other melanomas may start as a new pigmented lesion that starts to grow in a normal area of the skin. Most melanomas are irregular in shape with uneven areas raised above the skin, although some may grow just below the skin and be felt as a hard nodule. Many melanomas are dark brown or even black in color, but some may be reddish or blue in color, and others may even be flesh colored. Some melanomas may develop areas of bleeding, a process referred to as ulceration.

I am suspicious, then, that it may be melanoma when I see a mole change in appearance or begin to bleed, or the development of a new pigmented skin lesion in a previously normal area of skin.

Please remember that most skin growths, or lesions, are *not* melanoma, and are not even cancerous. Furthermore, of all skin cancers, only about 5 percent are melanoma. That is precisely why determining the source of skin cancers is so essential, since the non-melanoma cancers are more easily treated and the diagnosis of melanoma warrants more attention. Even though the odds favor a benign skin lesion, always try to find out as soon as possible that a new growth or a change in a known mole definitely is not melanoma: *Early recognition saves lives.*

Where is Melanoma Found on the Body?

Melanoma can occur anywhere that melanocytes, the pigment-producing cells of the body, are found. The most common location is the skin, and melanomas arising in the skin are referred to as *cutaneous melanomas*. As I mentioned, they may occur within an existing mole or may start in a previously normal-appearing part of the skin.

Table 1-4. Distribution of cutaneous melanoma

Skin site	Frequency
Head and neck	22–43%
Chest, abdomen, and back	13–32%
Arms	17–23%
Legs	21–25%
Unknown	2%

Melanomas may also occur in the mucous membranes around the mouth and nasal cavities (called *mucosal melanomas*) or around the anus (called *anal melanomas*). Another form of melanoma, called *ocular melanoma*, can even develop in the eye and is, in fact, the most common tumor of the eye. (Because they do not behave exactly like cutaneous or skin melanomas, mucosal, anal, and ocular melanomas are discussed separately in Chapter 9.)

After a melanoma has spread to other internal organs or lymph nodes, the original site cannot always be identified. Experts believe that, in such cases, the immune system may have destroyed the original (or primary) melanoma.

Table 1-5. Sites of melanoma on the body

Body site	Frequency of melanoma
Skin	92%
Eye	5%
Mucous membranes	2%
Unknown	1%

Who Gets Melanoma?

Melanoma is not a disease of the elderly. Most patients are diagnosed during their forties or fifties. Very rarely, melanoma has been reported in young infants (see the age distribution of melanoma in Figure 1-1). Race is an important filter, as melanoma most commonly strikes Caucasians of European descent. The disease is less prevalent among African Americans and is very rare in the Japanese population. Nonetheless, melanoma can and does occur in nearly all races and can be found all over the world.

Melanoma is strongly associated with exposure to the sun, especially for Caucasians. Proximity to the equator also increases your risk of melanoma. The highest risk of melanoma in the world occurs in Australia, where the disease affects 1 in every 60 Australians. Although nothing has been proven yet, this striking increase in melanoma may be related to the degradation of the protective ozone layer (which shields out harmful ultraviolet light), combined with the popularity of sunbathing and outdoor activities.

A familial or genetic form of melanoma is responsible for approximately 10 percent of all melanoma cases. The next chapter explains the causes and additional risk factors for developing melanoma.

Percentage of Reported Melanoma Cases in the United States

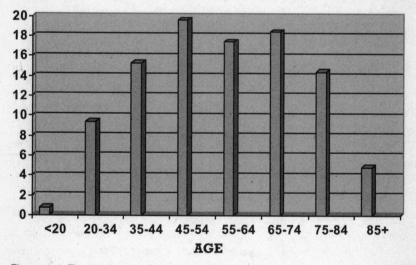

Figure 1-1. The distribution of melanoma by age

Based on data from the National Cancer Institute SEER Cancer Statistics Review, 1975–2001.

Why Is Melanoma So Dangerous?

When a melanoma is confined to the skin, it is usually treated easily by surgical removal. If melanoma grows to a certain depth within the dermis, however, some cells may break off and spread. These renegade cells usually enter the lymphatic system in the dermis and spread to nearby lymph nodes. From there they may spread almost anywhere else in the body, where they can cause serious damage to other organs and threaten life.

Although malignant melanoma accounts for only about 5 percent of all skin cancers, it is responsible for about 80 percent of all deaths related to skin cancer. In the United States, an estimated 52,000 people develop melanoma annually; almost 8,000 people die of melanoma each year, or twenty people every day. Melanoma is the sixth leading cause of cancer-related deaths in men and the seventh leading cause of cancer-related deaths in women. Melanoma has become the leading cause of cancer deaths in women between the ages of twenty-five and thirty.

Melanoma is also increasing at a faster rate than almost any other cancer. In 1935 melanoma afflicted 1 of every 1,500 persons living in the United States. This rate has steadily increased by 5–7 percent per year, so that by the year 2000 melanoma struck one in every seventy-five persons. The true incidence of melanoma may be much higher, since many skin lesions are destroyed by freezing, laser ablation, and other methods where biopsy confirmation of melanoma is not obtained or reported.

Although this data may sound disturbing, there is some good news: Despite the soaring number of melanoma cases, *the mortality rate has not increased proportionately during the last twenty years*. This may be due to the fact that melanoma is being detected earlier, when it is more likely to be cured, or it may be that better surgical techniques are achieving better cure rates.

In the next few chapters you will learn more about the causes of melanoma and how to prevent the disease, how to identify melanoma, and current treatment options and experimental therapies being developed for patients with melanoma.

Columbia Melanoma Center Case Studies

A thirty-two-year-old medical resident named Juan was working at the hospital when he noticed a dark, pigmented skin lesion on his left great toe, which had increased in size for about three months. Originally from Puerto Rico, he had spent a lot of time in the sun but there was no melanoma in his family. When I examined Juan, I found a one-centimeter smooth, flat blue-black pigmented lesion over the upper part of his toe. There was no evidence of abnormal lymph nodes in the leg or groin. We performed an excision of the skin lesion using a local anesthetic. After the pathologist reported that the lesion was a blue nevus and the margins of the lesion were all normal skin, I was able to reassure Juan that this was not melanoma. I advised him to have his dermatologist do at least an annual checkup, sooner if he notices any other unusual skin lesions.

This case is typical of pigmented skin lesions. The change in the size of the lesion over a three-month period was the most worrisome sign and the reason Juan was referred for evaluation. Like most people's pigmented skin lesions, his turned out to be of no serious consequence. The pathology report confirmed that the lesion was benign and the excision provided adequate treatment for Juan. Although I might have chosen to simply observe the skin lesion and remove it later, the recent change in size and Juan's peace of mind made me opt for excision.

Ask Your Doctor

If you develop a new skin lesion or notice a change in an old skin mole, ask the following questions:

1. *Is the lesion pigmented or non-pigmented?* Pigmented lesions are usually brown or black and are more worrisome for melanoma than non-pigmented lesions.
2. *Is the lesion suspicious for malignancy or cancer?* Many doctors will have experience looking at skin lesions and may be able to tell you what the problem is by simple inspection.

3. *Should I see a dermatologist?* A dermatologist is a doctor who has additional training in diseases of the skin and may be better equipped to identify difficult lesions. Many dermatologists are also trained in the treatment of skin cancers.

4. *Do I need a biopsy?* A biopsy is the only way to be certain of what the lesion is. It must be examined by a trained pathologist with experience in skin diseases. Always ask that your doctor review the pathology report with you after any biopsy procedure.

5. *Is my family at risk for developing a skin lesion or cancer?* Some types of skin cancer, especially melanoma, may be more common in close relatives. If your doctor believes that you have this type of cancer, it may be helpful to have close family members (parents, children, and siblings) see a dermatologist for a routine examination or screening so that lesions can be detected as early as possible.

CHAPTER TWO

What Causes Melanoma?

YOU NOW KNOW that melanoma is a type of skin cancer that occurs when the normal melanocytes divide without control. But what causes those normal melanocytes to divide so quickly and chaotically? What makes the melanoma cells then spread from the skin to the internal organs? Exactly what causes melanoma? The more we know about the causes of melanoma, the closer we may be to preventing melanoma from occurring in the first place. Scientists have already uncovered at least some factors that may confer a higher risk of developing melanoma. Certain risk factors can be controlled—how much and how often the skin is exposed to sunlight, for example. Other risk factors, such as genetic makeup, cannot be controlled. Even in the case of genetic risk, however, the more we know, the better armed we are to combat melanoma through early identification of those at higher risk for the disease.

Risk Factors You Can Control: Your Environment

The major cause of any cancer is a mutation, or change, in the DNA of a particular cell type. In the case of melanoma, the cell is the melanocyte. It stands to reason that anything changing the DNA of the melanocyte cell may result in abnormal melanocyte growth and

eventually cancer. So let's look at environmental factors that may nega-
tively affect the DNA of melanocyte cells.

Sun Exposure

It probably comes as no surprise that the single greatest risk factor
for developing melanoma is exposure to the sun. (Very recent work in
genetics may change the hierarchy of risk factors in the near future,
however.) Sunlight contains two invisible rays beyond violet in the spectrum: ultraviolet A and ultraviolet B rays. These ultraviolet rays, a type
of radiation derived from the energy in the sun, can burn the skin. In addition to the sun, ultraviolet radiation is also found in sunlamps and tanning booths. The ultraviolet B rays are more likely than the A rays to
cause sunburns; and it has been well documented that when experimental
mice are exposed to ultraviolet B, they develop melanoma. There is evidence that when melanocyte cells are exposed to ultraviolet B rays, their
DNA is damaged and they lose the ability to repair it. Once this happens, the melanocyte is unable to control its own growth, which you
may recall is the beginning of cancer. The reason why we think ultraviolet B rays are an especially important risk factor in the development
of melanoma and other skin cancers is because of their sunburning
ability.

Although the ultraviolet A rays are less likely to burn, these rays can
penetrate into deeper layers of the skin. Many scientists now believe that
ultraviolet A rays may cause melanoma at worst and premature aging of
the skin at best.

While clouds screen out the visible part of sunlight, the ultraviolet
rays are usually not deflected and may reach exposed areas of the skin
even when it is not sunny out. The ultraviolet A and B rays from the sun
are strongest in the summer months and from around 10 AM until 2 PM
most days. The best way to avoid ultraviolet radiation is to stay out of
the sun during these peak hours.

The well-established role of sun exposure in causing melanoma may
be less important than the genetic factors that are present in some peo-

ple. If you know you have genetic markers or a family history of melanoma, then avoiding excessive sunlight can be a powerful way to help reduce your risk of a melanoma.

Perhaps more significant than the mere fact of exposure to the sun is how your particular skin reacts to sunlight. Some people develop slow tans over time when they lie out on the beach all day. Others are severely burned within a few hours. How the sun affects your skin may be an even more important risk factor than the total time of exposure to sunlight. People who tend to sunburn more quickly are at a greater risk for melanoma than those who tan easily or whose skin is relatively unaffected by sun exposure.

The Childhood Time Element

Another melanoma risk factor is the amount of time spent in the sun during childhood, particularly between the ages of ten and twenty-four. The reasons for this are not entirely clear. Some scientists believe that childhood is a period when kids are more likely to participate in outdoor activities. Because it takes years for sun damage to accumulate and cause a melanoma, other scientists think that those individuals who are in the sun at an earlier age—which equals a longer total time of exposure—are more at risk. Whatever the reasons, a person who has a history of severe sunburns as a child or teenager is at an especially high risk for the development of melanoma. Even just one or two such bad sunburns can increase the risk of melanoma in later life. I always ask patients about their youthful sun exposure if they are concerned about their chances of getting melanoma.

Geography

The sun is naturally stronger at the equator than at the North or South Pole; therefore, you might conclude that people who live closer to the equator would be at higher risk for melanoma. You'd be only partially right. Caucasians with light and fair skin do appear to be at a high risk for melanoma if they live closer to the equator. Australia, which lies close to the equator and has a large proportion of Caucasian inhabitants, also has the highest incidence of melanoma in the world. One of every sixty Australians develops melanoma. Other countries near the equator, however, do not have such a high incidence of melanoma. The reason may be that dark-skinned individuals, such as most Africans who live near the equator, are protected from melanoma. While there is evidence that dark-skinned individuals produce more skin pigments that help protect them from melanoma, there may also be genetic factors that guard against melanoma. Our most reasonable conclusion is that the geographic risk for melanoma is highest for Caucasian people living near the equator.

Other Possibilities

Occasionally people develop melanoma on parts of the body, such as the feet or buttocks, not commonly exposed to the sun. We think that genetic or other unknown factors must play a major role in these cases.

One potentially fruitful line of inquiry involved viruses. After all, viruses often infect specific cells and disrupt the cell's DNA. While a great deal of attention has been focused on determining if viruses can cause cancer, to date it's been very difficult to prove for most human cancers. There are several examples of viruses causing cancer in animals, such as the feline leukemia virus that causes leukemia in cats. We know of at least three human cancers definitely caused by viral infections. The Epstein-Barr virus causes a rare cancer of the nasal passages, found in Africans. Kaposi's sarcoma—an AIDS-related cancer—is associated with a recently discovered herpes virus. A specific type of human papilloma virus is linked to cancer of the cervix in women. Although there is no definitive evidence for a virus being involved in melanoma, there have been some reports in the medical literature of melanoma cells containing a type of human papilloma virus that is known to cause skin warts. This may be a simple coincidence—or it may prove to have a role in the development of melanoma.

KNOWN ENVIRONMENTAL RISK FACTORS FOR MELANOMA
- Sun exposure (especially easy burning in sun)
- Time outdoors (especially during childhood)
- Proximity to equator (especially in light-skinned individuals)
- Viruses (possibly human papilloma virus)

Risk Factors You Cannot Control: Your Genetics

Over the last ten years it has become clear that genetic factors are responsible for many cases of melanoma and may be even more important than sun exposure or other environmental factors. The presence of a genetic risk factor does not mean you have to throw up your hands in despair, thinking that there is nothing you can do. On the contrary, determining you are at increased risk through genetic factors indicates that you might benefit from more frequent screening so that any melanoma can be identified as early as possible, when it is completely curable. Of course, anyone with a genetic risk factor needs to be on the alert and pay careful attention to controlling environmental factors, most notably sun exposure.

There are two ways to evaluate your genetic risk for melanoma, one simple and inexpensive, the other costly and more complex. First, there are some easy-to-identify high-risk genetic factors that may make people prone to developing melanoma. I will discuss these below in detail. Then, I will explain how genetic testing, a more ambiguous method in some ways, can pinpoint abnormalities in genes related to melanoma.

Red Flags

Previous Melanoma or Family History

The most obvious risk factor for melanoma is having had a melanoma in the past. Most melanomas can be identified early and easily cured, but once melanoma has occurred there is as much as a nine hundred-fold increased risk for developing a second melanoma. If you are a melanoma survivor, it is critical that you avoid any environmental risks and go for regular skin screening since your chances of developing a new melanoma are very high.

Although not as significant as a previous melanoma, a family history of melanoma is also a risk factor. The closer the relative, the higher the risk. Serious attention to melanoma prevention and screening is certainly called for if your parent, sibling, or child has ever been diagnosed. Grandparents are not considered first-degree relatives. In most cases the genetic links in families are unknown or vague, but there are syndromes in which the genes involved have been clearly defined, and I will describe the familial melanoma syndromes separately.

Previous Skin Cancers

Basal cell carcinoma and squamous cell carcinoma, much more common than melanoma, are types of skin cancer that are not usually considered serious. There is some evidence, however, that people with these other skin cancers may be at a higher risk for melanoma. We do not really understand why this is the case, although it may relate to a general abnormal skin response to sun damage. In fact, some reports suggest that there maybe a seventeen-fold higher risk of melanoma in people who have had other types of skin cancer. So, once a skin cancer of any type develops, it means regular lifelong screening for melanoma is essential.

Moles

The number of moles you have is genetically determined, as I've mentioned. The presence of many large moles (nevi) is a strong risk factor for melanoma; the risk increases threefold in people who have five or more moles measuring greater than five millimeters in diameter. Whenever a mole changes its size, shape, or appearance there is an increased chance for melanoma. If a mole looks different in any way—even if it appears to be getting smaller or shrinking—it warrants a trip to the doctor for evaluation. Large moles, particularly those larger than about five millimeters, or the size of a silver dollar, are more likely to harbor melanoma. Likewise, the more moles someone has, the greater the melanoma risk.

The type of mole also affects your risk of melanoma. As you know, melanoma occurs when melanocytes grow uncontrollably due to changes in their DNA. However, long before the melanocyte becomes a melanoma, its DNA may change in subtle ways but enough to alter the cells. These subtly altered cells are called *dysplastic* by pathologists, and we call such moles dysplastic, or atypical, nevi. Usually a dysplastic nevus is larger than five millimeters in diameter, contains variable areas of coloration, may be irregular in appearance on the skin, or has indistinct borders. These nevi, found in 5–7 percent of the entire Caucasian population, occur in almost 40 percent of patients with melanoma and therefore represent a strong risk factor for melanoma. When a large number of dysplastic nevi are found in a person or family members, I immediately suspect a familial (or inherited) form of melanoma.

Freckles

Referred to as ephelides by medical professionals, freckles are common tan skin blemishes. Like moles, they are genetically determined and are more prevalent in fair-skinned and light-haired individuals. Freckles usually occur in multiple numbers on areas of the skin exposed to the sun. Most freckles first appear around two years of age and may increase in number through young adulthood but then begin to fade. In some cases they may be more noticeable during times of significant sun exposure, such as the summer months. Freckles are due to the skin's melanocytes reacting to ultraviolet A and B rays by producing more melanin in genetically predisposed individuals. While freckles by themselves are not considered dangerous, there is some evidence that people with a strong freckling tendency may also be at increased risk of melanoma.

Skin and Hair Color

The genes that we inherit from our parents determine a number of skin features over which we have no control. Inherited skin traits may determine the risk of melanoma. People with lighter skin, such as Caucasians, have a much higher risk of melanoma than dark-skinned individuals. Those with olive skin appear to have a risk for melanoma in between light- and dark-skinned individuals, suggesting that skin color is a fairly reliable, albeit small, predictor of risk. In general, light skin confers only about a two-fold increased risk of melanoma over olive or black skin.

Similar to skin color, hair color may also predict melanoma risk. The highest risk occurs in people with red hair, who have about a three-fold increased risk compared to brown- or black-haired individuals. Blond hair confers about a one-and-a-half fold increased risk. Although you cannot change the skin or hair color you were born with, you can be more cautious about melanoma if you are light skinned with red or blond hair.

The Immune System

If your immune system is weakened, you may be more prone to developing melanoma. One possible reason may be the inability of a compromised immune system to destroy melanoma cells. People who have had transplants and require immune suppressive medication, those with genetic disorders of the immune system, and HIV-infected individuals all have an increased risk for both benign nevi and melanoma. The degree of risk correlates with how badly and for how long the immune system is suppressed. Children who had kidney transplants at an early age are more prone to melanoma than adults who have kidney transplants, for example. The risk of non-melanoma skin cancer is actually much higher than the risk of melanoma. But when melanoma does occur, it is often very advanced and much more difficult to treat than in patients with a normal immune system. All patients with weakened immune systems, no matter the cause, need to have frequent, careful skin examinations.

KNOWN GENETIC RISK FACTORS FOR MELANOMA
- Prior melanoma
- Family history of melanoma
- Non-melanoma skin cancer
- Changing mole
- Presence of many large moles
- Freckling tendency
- Race (especially Caucasian)
- Skin color
- Hair color
- Immunosuppression states

Familial Syndromes

Most cases of melanoma develop in people without any history of melanoma or any family members with melanoma. This is referred to as sporadic melanoma and currently accounts for close to 90 percent of all melanoma cases. However, 10 percent of melanoma is related to inherited genetic disorders and is called familial melanoma. The differences between sporadic and familial melanoma are listed in Table 2-1. In general, sporadic melanoma tends to occur in slightly older individuals and is characterized by a single melanoma in a person without any family members having melanoma. Some of these patients will have a dysplastic nevus, a mole that has changed and is thought to be a precursor to melanoma. In contrast, familial melanoma occurs in younger people, may often involve more than one melanoma at diagnosis, and a history of melanoma in at least two close relatives. Familial melanoma is nearly always associated with the presence of dysplastic nevi, but in familial cases dysplastic nevi occur on parts of the skin not exposed to the sun, whereas in sporadic cases of melanoma these nevi are more likely to be on sun-exposed areas. Familial melanoma is inherited, as one or more genetic defects are passed from parent to child. You have familial melanoma syndrome if you meet at least three of the criteria in Table 2-1.

Table 2-1. Differences between sporadic melanoma and familial melanoma

Feature	Sporadic Melanoma	Familial Melanoma
Age at diagnosis	Older; average age, 54	Younger; average age, 35
Number of melanomas	Usually 1	May be more than 1
Dysplastic nevi present	Some people	Most people
Family history of melanoma	No	2 or more first degree relatives

Dysplastic Nevus Syndrome

Of the inherited familial syndromes, we know the most about dysplastic nevus syndrome, which is responsible for 5–10 percent of all cases of melanoma and is characterized by the presence of many dysplastic nevi. Some dysplastic nevus syndrome patients have over one hundred nevi. The syndrome is inherited in a dominant manner: there is a 50:50 chance that an affected person will pass it on to his or her child. Even though the dysplastic nevi identify people at risk for melanoma, the actual melanoma may occur in previously normal areas of the skin, rather than directly on the dysplastic nevus. This is why we do not always remove every nevus, but only those that are new or show signs of changing in the recent past. The relationship between the nevi and the melanoma is not entirely clear. Therefore, individuals with dysplastic nevus syndrome require careful skin examination to identify suspicious nevi or new skin lesions, and early removal is recommended. These individuals are considered to have a familial form of melanoma, and screening or genetic testing of close relatives should be considered.

The specific genetic defects in patients with dysplastic nevus syndrome are beginning to be defined. Many of the genes play a role in the coordination of cell division, a process referred to as the *cell cycle* in melanocyte cells. Defects in the CDK4 gene, involved in the control of the cell cycle, have been reported in at least three families affected with this syndrome. Abnormalities of the CDKN2a gene, also involved in cell cycle control, have been seen in 20 percent of tested families with the syndrome. Children of a parent with a known genetic defect can be tested for that genetic defect.

Xeroderma Pigmentosa

Xeroderma pigmentosa is another rare inherited disorder in which affected individuals lack the enzymes that repair DNA in skin cells exposed to ultraviolet radiation. The disease occurs in one patient for every 250,000 people in the general population. In most people, damage caused by the ultraviolet radiation can be repaired, but with xeroderma pigmentosa the repair enzymes are defective, so the ultraviolet damage accumulates more quickly. The result is an increased risk of skin cancer, including melanoma. The skin cancers in these individuals often occur at a very young age, even less than five years old, and so affected people must avoid sun exposure and have frequent skin examinations to identify skin cancer or melanoma as early as possible. Most people with xeroderma pigmentosa ultimately die from melanoma or skin cancer, often before the age of twenty. There are genetic tests available for this rare disease and testing of the amniotic fluid is possible in pregnant women. Women with a family history of xeroderma pigmentosa may consider this test, although there is a slight risk to the pregnancy due to the collection of amniotic fluid.

Genetic Testing for Melanoma Markers

The revolution in molecular biology and the ability of scientists to study genes has led to new and unexpected findings for a number of diseases, including melanoma. Melanoma strikes when the DNA of melanocytes in the skin mutates, making them apt to grow out of control and spread to internal organs. Most cancer researchers believe that this process is due to the loss of specific genes that control the start and stop of cell division and growth. More recently they have identified a number of genes that stop cells from dividing and may even cause injured cells to die, in a process called *apoptosis*. This cell death is a normal body function that destroys injured, stressed, or abnormal cells and makes room for new normal cells. In melanoma, as well as other cancers, apoptosis is unable to occur, as the genes that regulate the cell death are lost or damaged. Scientists have isolated many of these genes by comparing the DNA in melanoma cells with the DNA in normal melanocytes.

Genes are composed of segments of DNA; individual genes are organized into groups on each chromosome; chromosomes also are comprised of some DNA whose function is not known. Humans have forty-six chromosomes, all of which contain the genes that determine the properties of every cell. Now that the whole DNA sequence of human chromosomes has been mapped, the discovery of abnormal DNA in individual genes has become much easier. Before this information was available, a powerful tool for identifying abnormal genes in melanoma cells was to compare the chromosomes of normal melanocytes and melanoma cells. Scientists could often find abnormal areas of a specific chromosome in melanoma cells when they compared them to the normal melanocyte. Investigators would then try to determine which genes are located at the sites of the discovered mutation: the very cause of the melanocyte's destructive behavior. Once a particular gene is identified, scientists can see if the same gene is defective in other melanoma cells. Interestingly, most of the defective genes are responsible for cell growth or cell death, which explains why these cells may not be able to regulate their growth. If you look at the frequency of these defects in melanoma cells, you can see that not all melanoma cells have the same genetic defects. This suggests that there may be some subtle differences in melanoma from person to person and why some melanomas respond to treatment better than others.

The outcome of this research may be a double-edged sword, since we can now test for genetic defects that identify people who may be at risk for melanoma—even before they develop the disease. As of this writing, genetic tests that measure chromosomal damage in melanocytes and specific gene mutations, such as the p16^{INK4} gene on chromosome 9, can be conducted. The p16^{INK4} gene controls the growth rate of melanoma cells and is abnormal in about 32–46 percent of all melanomas. The fact that the gene is *not* present in 54–68 percent of melanoma patients underscores the potential problems inherent in genetic testing. Individuals may have a normal test for this gene but still be at risk for melanoma due to defects in other genes. Genetic tests must be interpreted very carefully to avoid either a false sense of complacency or out-of-proportion panic. If the test is positive, there is definitely a risk of melanoma and you will no doubt want regular screening. If the test is normal, however, you may still need screening since other genes may be involved. This is true for most genetic tests of cancer. Genetic testing requires consultation with a genetic counselor familiar with the test, the implications of positive and negative results, the psychological and legal implications of testing, and plans for screening pending the results of testing.

Identification of individual genetic changes requires a separate blood test, and so the length of time required varies depending on how many genes are being tested at a time. The tests are expensive, but in certain cases—notably breast cancer—testing has saved lives. Still, genetic testing for disease remains controversial.

We are at an early stage of genetic testing and our ability to use these tests effectively may become better delineated in the future. At present, I rarely rely on genetic tests of my patients, but prefer to consider all of the other risk factors. I advise people who may be at risk to avoid sun exposure, use appropriate protection if they must be in the sun, and to have regular skin examinations. In addition, I teach self-examination since early detection and removal of a suspicious mole or melanoma can lead to complete cure. The possibility of replacing abnormal genes for melanoma, which I explain in Chapter 14, remains purely experimental at this time. I consider genetic testing only when there is a strong family history with at least two close relatives with melanoma and when the family understands the limitations of genetic test results.

Columbia Melanoma Center Case Studies

James was a fifty-six-year-old man with a long history of multiple dysplastic nevi when he came to see me. He had no other medical problems but said he had been a lifeguard as a teenager and burned easily in the sun. When I examined him, I saw he had many nevi, scattered especially over his arms and upper chest. His local dermatologist had removed several lesions, starting when James was thirty years old. At age thirty-six he had a very early melanoma removed from his arm. Six months before coming to the Melanoma Center he noticed that a nevus on his chest had become darker and larger. It turned out to be a malignant melanoma, and he had it excised. His concern for his two children, thirteen and seventeen years old, prompted his appointment with me. They both have multiple freckles and light complexions, so James wanted to know whether they should have genetic testing, and how they should be evaluated to determine their risk for melanoma.

I was certain that James had the dysplastic nevus syndrome because of his history of multiple dysplastic nevi and melanomas at a relatively young age. Although it is not unusual to develop a second melanoma—even twenty years later—this scenario made it more likely to be a case of familial melanoma and his children, who had inherited his light complexion and tendency to burn in the sun, may be at increased risk for melanoma also. We discussed the increased risk of melanoma in the children and decided to have them come to the Melanoma Center for a routine skin screening examination. I counseled both children on ways to avoid sun and ultraviolet radiation exposure and advised that they have an annual skin examination to identify any dysplastic nevi and to remove any suspicious lesions. We also discussed the benefits and risks of genetic testing for the children, but decided against it, since our plan would not change no matter what the test results showed.

Ask Your Doctor

If you are worried that you might be at risk for melanoma or a familial syndrome, ask the following questions:

1. *Do I have many dysplastic nevi?* The presence of freckles or moles does not necessarily mean that you have dysplastic nevi. If there is any doubt about a particular mole the doctor should have it removed to determine its nature with certainty.

2. *Do you consider me to be at risk for melanoma?* Most primary physicians and dermatologists will be able to determine your risk for melanoma based on your medical history and physical examination. The best way to beat melanoma is to prevent it in the first place, so you can also ask for advice on melanoma prevention (I detail how to prevent melanoma in Chapter 3).

3. *Should I see a dermatologist?* A dermatologist has additional training in diseases of the skin and can often help recognize people at risk for melanoma and recommend preventive measures.

4. *Should I have a genetic test for melanoma?* There are benefits and risks of genetic testing and whether to have a test is something you should discuss with your personal physician and a genetic counselor. Think about what you will do if the test shows that you have the gene that increases the risk of melanoma. Also consider what you will do if you do not have the gene. It is possible that testing could lead to a false sense of security, since other potentially harmful genes may be present that are not part of the test. Consider what effect the test may have on other members of your family and ask them if they want to know the results.

5. *How often should I see a dermatologist to have my skin examined?* This is an important question and the answer depends on your risk of developing melanoma. For those at low risk, an examination once a year is sufficient. If you already have had a melanoma, a professional screening every six months is standard. If you have a genetic disorder or a syndrome such as xeroderma pigmentosa, then screening may need to occur even more frequently.

6. *At what age should skin screening begin?* Although there is little evidence for defining the best age to start skin screening, the answer depends on how great the risk of developing melanoma is for an individual. In families with a known melanoma history, screening should be considered as early as five years old. If a child has extensive or unusual moles, screening should start as soon as possible.

CHAPTER THREE

Can We Prevent Melanoma?

TODAY, MOST SCIENTISTS believe that a mutation in the DNA of melanocyte cells results in melanoma. The DNA mutation, in turn, occurs in certain genes and cancer researchers have even identified some specific genetic changes responsible for melanoma. Yet there still is nothing precise enough to claim as an exact cause. The closer we get to pinpointing the cause, the closer we are to preventing melanoma. But we are not quite there yet: There still is no *proven* way to prevent melanoma.

There is, however, a way to prevent melanoma from spreading aggressively and becoming life threatening. As I've said before and will continue to emphasize throughout this book, *it is crucial to recognize melanoma as early as possible*. In its earliest stages it can be treated easily and effectively by simple removal. Careful, regular examination of the skin is the single best way to find melanoma early on. Such an examination is also referred to as *screening*. Either a professional, such as a dermatologist, can perform it, or you can check for skin cancer on yourself, using the Early Detection Self-Exam and Body Map, which I'll describe below. In addition, I explain some strategies that involve sun avoidance and using sunscreen when you can't avoid the sun.

Again, any suspicious lesions should be evaluated by a melanoma specialist who can determine if a biopsy is indicated. The good news is that most pesky moles will be nothing, but for those at risk for melanoma early detection is the best way to survive the disease.

Avoiding Sun Exposure

We cannot currently change the risk factors that put us at risk for developing melanoma. Therefore, most efforts in prevention focus on avoiding those environmental factors that add to the threat of melanoma. The most important of these factors is exposure to sunlight. The amount of time that people are exposed to sunlight—the ultraviolet A and B rays in particular—clearly determines the actual risk of melanoma. The best method for avoiding harmful ultraviolet radiation is to avoid contact with sunlight as much as is possible or practical. Common sense should prevail. Exposure to ultraviolet radiation is most damaging during the summer months between the hours of about 10 AM and 2 PM. During these hours, approximately two-thirds of the entire day's ultraviolet rays reach the Earth. Consequently, people at significant risk of melanoma should try to avoid outdoor activities during these times.

The ultraviolet (UV) index is used to measure, or forecast, the amount of ultraviolet rays expected to reach the Earth's surface when the sun is highest in the sky. It will depend on the location of the sun on a particular day, the presence of clouds, the amount of ozone over the site, and the altitude of the city. The UV index is reported as a number from 0–10, and the higher the number the faster the ultraviolet rays will cause damage to the skin (see Table 3-1). The UV index is usually reported in the daily newspaper or as part of many television weather reports. The UV index can also be found for fifty-eight cities at the National Weather Service Web site: www.cpc.ncep.noaa.gov/products /stratosphere/uv_index/uv_current.html.

Whenever the UV index is 5 or greater you should consider some sort of sun protection even if your risk of melanoma is low.

Table 3-1. The UV Index and exposure levels

UV Index	Exposure Level
<2	Low
3–5	Moderate
6–7	High
8–10	Very High
11+	Extreme

I am often asked about the best way to protect the skin if you cannot avoid the sun. If you absolutely must be outdoors, then seek out a shaded area and wear clothing that covers as much of your skin as possible. Don't forget a hat for your head, which is also vulnerable, and ultraviolet-protection sunglasses to protect the eyes. Although hair provides some added protection from the sun, the ultraviolet rays can still damage the skin under hair and we know that bald spots are especially prone to skin cancer and melanoma. Melanocytes are present in and around the eyes, so it is also possible to get melanoma of the eye. Therefore, a hat and protective sunglasses are always a good idea.

A shirt with long sleeves and long pants provide better protection than any form of sunscreen or sunblock. There is some evidence that different fabrics may provide differing levels of protection from ultraviolet rays. The amount of protection probably depends on the fiber content, the thickness of the fiber, and the type of knit or weave used. But there is not enough information at the present time to recommend any particular type of clothing as better or worse for protecting the skin against the sun's harmful rays.

If you must work outdoors and cannot schedule the hours that you are outside, definitely adopt all the strategies I mention above.

*   *   *

PERHAPS EVEN MORE important than avoiding the sun as an adult is keeping time in the sun to a minimum for children. The risk of melanoma seems to be highest in children exposed to excessive sunlight during childhood. A few studies suggest that two or more serious sunburns during childhood are a strong predictor of melanoma in adulthood. Prevention really needs to begin during infancy; babies and young children should be monitored to make sure they are not left under the sun for long periods of time. This is especially important if they tend to burn rather than tan after being in the sun. Sun protection should be taken seriously in children with any of the listed risk factors shown below. Recently, the American Academy of Pediatrics endorsed the use of sunscreen in infants and children as a safe way to prevent sun damage and possible skin cancer.

RISK FACTORS FOR MELANOMA IN CHILDREN
- One or more sunburns
- Melanoma in close relatives
- Spends much time outdoors
- Fair skin complexion
- Large number of moles
- Large number of freckles
- Known hereditary syndrome in family

The risk of exposure to ultraviolet rays also depends on where you live: The closer to the equator, the stronger the sun's ultraviolet radiation. Light-skinned individuals should be especially cautious if they live or travel to parts of the world with high levels of sunlight. Another significant geographic feature that may surprise you in terms of sun exposure is elevation. In general the sun's rays are about 5 percent stronger for every 1,000 feet in elevation above sea level. In Denver, Colorado, which is a mile above sea level, the sun's rays are about 25 percent stronger than they are in Richmond, Virginia, for example.

What About Sunscreen?

By now, I think everyone, at least in this country, knows that the medical community strongly advises wearing sunscreen. But such a blanket decree still leaves many questions, and patients, friends, and family often ask me about sunscreen. Exactly what *is* sunscreen? How effective is sunscreen? What are the best products? What's the difference between sunscreen and sunblock? What is the SPF and which SPF should I use? Do I really need to wear it every day, even in winter? These are a few of the most common inquiries.

Sunscreen, which was first developed and sold in 1944, is a general term for a substance that protects the skin from the dangerous ultraviolet rays found in sunlight. Sunscreen comes in the form of a cream, ointment, lotion, spray, or gel; to my knowledge there is no data as to whether the form makes any difference. Sunscreen works by reflecting, absorbing, or scattering the ultraviolet A and B rays so that they cannot penetrate into the skin. Many of the earlier sunscreen products only provided protection against ultraviolet B rays. The ozone layer provides protection largely against the ultraviolet A rays. For every 1 percent loss of the ozone layer there is an additional 1 percent increase in the development of melanoma. Therefore, you should make sure that the sunscreen you choose is effective against both ultraviolet A and B rays. Most sunscreen ingredients fall into two categories—physical or chemical agents. Physical agents include inorganic molecules, such as zinc or titanium, and these absorb ultraviolet rays. In fact, zinc oxide is probably one of the best overall blockers of ultraviolet rays and has been used for more than thirty years. The chemical agents are organic molecules with varying degrees of defense activity against ultraviolet A and B rays. Table 3-2 lists some of the commonly used ingredients in sunscreen and provides a list of how effective they are for ultraviolet A and B rays. If a product's label states it is "broad spectrum," it does contain active ingredients to block both ultraviolet A and B rays. Additional agents may help soothe the skin or have other non-medical effects but are not known to play a role in sun protection. One exception is anti-oxidants, which may help prevent skin damage.

Table 3-2. Selected agents used in sunscreen preparations

Classification	Agent	Ultraviolet Protection	Comments
Physical Agents	Zinc oxide	A and B rays	Most powerful agent
	Titanium oxide	B and some A rays	Not as effective as zinc oxide
Chemical Agents	Avobenzone (Parsol 1789)	A rays	Most effective agent for A rays
	Octyl dimethyl paba (PABA) and PABA esters	B rays only	
	Oxybenzone	B and some A rays	Provides moderate protection
	Dioxybenzone	B and some A rays	Similar to oxybenzone
	Red petrolatum	B and some A rays	Enhances the benzophenones
	Cinoxate	B rays only	Provides low protection
	Ethyl-p-methoxycinnamate	B rays only	Provides low protection
	Octyl methoxcinnamate (Octocrylene)	B rays only	Provides low protection
	Octyl salicylate	B rays	

CAN WE PREVENT MELANOMA?

Classification	Agent	Ultraviolet Protection	Comments
	Isopropyl dibenzoylmethane (Eusolex 8020)	A and B rays	Provides very high protection
	Menthyl anthranilate	A rays	
	Butyl methoxydibenzoylmethane	A rays	Not yet approved in the United States
Anti-oxidants	Vitamin C		May help prevent skin damage
	Vitamin E		May help prevent skin damage

The Sun Protection Factor, commonly abbreviated as SPF, is how products are rated on their degree of sunburn protection. The higher the SPF, the more protection it provides. When you have a fair complexion the sun will start to cause a burn in approximately ten minutes without protection. An SPF of 10 means that you can stay exposed to the sun ten times longer, or about one hundred minutes, before you will start to burn. So after one hundred minutes the risk of sunburn returns to the risk before the sunscreen was applied. If you use sunscreen SPF 30, your risk is reduced for three hundred minutes or five hours. When the SPF is less than 11 there is little protection and SPF levels between 12–29 only provide moderate protection. An SPF of 30 or greater is necessary to provide high enough protection against the ultraviolet rays. I recommend using an SPF of 30 or 45 for most of my patients. In addition, you should wear sunglasses with lenses that block at least 99 percent of the ultraviolet rays to shield your eyes. As for your lips, lip balm often includes sunblock, but melanoma of the lip is not common.

Try to apply sunscreen twenty to thirty minutes (but no earlier) be-

fore going outside. Deduct that amount of time from your total protection period. Use it whenever you go outdoors, even if the sun is not
shining, since the ultraviolet rays can get through the clouds even when
it's raining. If you're in the car, you don't need to be as vigilant: Rays do
not penetrate most glass. Reapply sunscreen every two to four hours depending on the SPF, no matter what activities you are engaged in. Reapply after going into any body of water, whether it's an ocean, lake, river,
swimming pool, or even if you're sweating in a sauna! Beware of products that state they are "waterproof." The FDA has not yet substantiated
the claim that sunscreen can be truly waterproof.

Sunscreen appears to be safe even when applied to infants under the
age of six months. Before applying sunscreen on young infants, test for
allergic reaction or irritation. Rub a small amount of sunscreen, around
the size of a dime, on the baby's upper back. If there is no reaction then
the product can be used safely. Although this trial and error approach
may seem bothersome, it is certainly worthwhile. The *Journal of the
American Medical Association* reported recently that children with freckles who wore SPF 30 sunscreen when they were outdoors had a 30–40
percent reduction in the number of new moles over a three-year period.
The American Academy of Pediatrics recently endorsed the use of sunscreen in infants and children of all ages. Check with your pediatrician
if you have any concern about using sunscreen on your children.

The use of sunscreen certainly protects your skin from premature aging and solar damage. There is also good evidence that the regular use
of sunscreen can prevent some forms of skin cancer, including basal cell
and squamous cell carcinomas. To date, however, there is no conclusive
evidence that sunscreen can prevent melanoma. While some doctors believe that sunscreen will protect against melanoma, not all studies agree
with this conclusion. The most recent large study, conducted in Europe
in 1995, divided over six hundred students into two groups. One group
was told to wear sunscreen whenever they went outside in the sun. The
second group was not given sunscreen. Both groups kept a log of how
much time they spent in the sun. After six months the investigators evaluated and examined both groups for evidence of new skin moles. They

found that those students who had been using the sunscreen actually spent more time in the sun and had more new moles to show for it. They concluded that sunscreen may give a false sense of security to people, who then spend more time than usual in the sun. Sunscreen use did not seem to prevent new moles and the authors of this study suggested that sunscreen may not protect against melanoma.

Although further studies are needed to better understand the role of sunscreen in melanoma prevention, for now it's reasonable to use sunscreen products. They do provide protection against other types of skin cancer, prevent premature skin aging, and ultimately may prove to protect against melanoma. Use sunscreen early and often. If you are at especially high risk of melanoma, avoid midday sun completely, use protective clothing, headgear, and sunglasses outside whenever possible, and use sunscreen for all other times when the skin or head cannot safely be covered.

You can still increase your risk of melanoma without ever setting foot outdoors. The same ultraviolet radiation found in the sun is generated from sunlamps and tanning booths. There is clear evidence that excessive tanning in salons is associated with melanoma as well as several other serious problems, such as premature skin aging, non-melanoma skin cancer, and cataracts. I always advise my patients to avoid tanning indoors as scrupulously as they avoid the sun outdoors. If you want to tan indoors despite this warning, do apply sunscreen and follow the same guidelines as for outdoor sun exposure.

Melanoma Screening

Screening for cancer is recommended when there is definite evidence that early detection changes the outcome for the patient, the screening procedure is easy to perform, and the screening is cost-effective. Melanoma screening satisfies all of these requirements. A large number of studies have been conducted in the United States, Europe, and especially Australia demonstrating that screening reduces the number of

advanced melanoma cases and may also influence survival. Yet neither patients nor physicians practice screening with any frequency. We
cannot currently predict which moles will turn into melanomas and we
know that some melanomas start in previously normal areas of the skin,
which is why a screening skin examination is indicated for all high risk
individuals. If there is any doubt as to degree of risk, then consider a
screening examination.

Avoiding sun exposure and using protective clothing and sunscreen
products are the only effective measures for reducing the chances of developing melanoma. Yet even these methods are no guarantee. That's
why early detection remains the single most important way to survive—
and live with—melanoma. In the next few chapters I will explain how
melanoma found at the early stages of the disease can be completely removed and the patient considered cured. But first I'll detail how to find
it early enough through the two primary techniques: professional skin
screening and self-examination, the procedures recommended by the
American Cancer Society.

Professional Skin Screening

A professional skin screening is usually performed by a board-certified
dermatologist—a doctor who has additional training in diseases of the
skin. Ask your dermatologist if he/she does this or if he/she can refer
you to a dermatologist who does. Infrequently, primary care physicians
or other health care professionals trained in the recognition and management of melanoma may offer screening as well. Ask your primary
doctor or dermatologist, "Do you perform screening for melanoma and
skin cancer?" In my experience most physicians are not taught this during their medical training and are usually happy to refer patients to
someone skilled in skin screening. The examination consists of a careful
visual inspection of the skin from the head (including under the hair) to
the bottom of the feet. Any suspicious lesions are noted and usually removed by a procedure called a biopsy (see Chapter 4). All of the moles
or other benign skin lesions are marked on a chart, similar to the one

shown in Figure 3-1. The height and width of larger lesions are measured and recorded on your medical chart. Then on follow-up screenings, the doctor can measure the lesions and compare the measurements from the previous screening. Any lesion that grows or changes can be detected easily. Some dermatologists take digital photographs of the skin, comparing photographs at each new visit to easily identify changes. I believe digital photography will become more and more affordable and I would certainly recommend searching out a doctor who is trained to do digital screening whenever possible.

How often should a professional screening be done? The schedule for screening depends on your risk factors. You and your doctor need to discuss this and come up with a plan. If a melanoma develops at any point, screening will no doubt happen more frequently. Likewise, if everything is normal for a few years, then screening can be done less often. If there is a small risk then I suggest screening once a year. If there is a significant risk of melanoma then screening should be done every six months. In some cases, such as patients with a history of aggressive melanoma or with an inherited syndrome, such as xeroderma pigmentosa, even more frequent screening may be recommended.

Early Detection Self-Exam and Body Map

The Early Detection Self-Exam is meant as an additional measure of protection to augment, not replace, the professional screening. It should be done in conjunction with a regular physician's evaluation. You know your body better than almost anyone else and will be able to determine small changes more readily—often before your appointment with the dermatologist.

The Early Detection Self-Exam should be performed once a month and is a good routine for everyone to develop. Follow the steps of the exam, detailed below, the same way each month. Pick an easy-to-remember date, such as the first of the month, or some other monthly occurrence that will jog your memory—pay day, poker night, a committee meeting. If you find something that does not seem normal, call your doctor or dermatologist immediately and have them check the area of concern. Often it is nothing and your mind can be put at ease. In a worst case scenario, it is suspicious. Then early biopsy or removal can be done and you may be saving your own life.

When should you start to perform skin examinations? Should you teach your children to do the exam? At what age should children begin? These are questions that we simply do not have good answers for yet. I certainly believe that children should be examined or instructed on how to perform a skin exam in high-risk families. If a brother, sister, or parent has had melanoma early screening is indicated. Keep in mind that screening is a positive way to prevent serious disease and find melanoma early when it is easier to cure. Tell your children the reasons for doing this examination and make sure that their concerns and questions are adequately addressed.

Begin the Early Detection Self-Exam just after taking a bath or shower. Stand in front of a full-length mirror and use a hand-held mirror for hard-to-see areas of the body. Examine yourself with a specific routine, going over the surface of the skin the same way every time. I suggest you start at the scalp and examine under the hair and areas around the hair. You may need to part your hair to see the entire scalp and use a comb or hair dryer to move hair out of the way. Use your fingertips to feel the scalp, which should be smooth. Many suspicious lesions are elevated off the surface of the skin and are more easily detected through touch than by eye due to hair obscuring the scalp.

Next, move to the face. Give special attention to the ears since small lesions may be difficult to see but are especially important to identify, as they are aggressive. Examine the cheeks, nostrils, eyelids, and neck in a systematic fashion.

Work downward from the neck to the shoulders, chest, abdomen, and genitalia. If you are a woman, be sure to lift up your breasts and examine the skin normally hidden from view since this is a common site for melanoma to hide. Once you've checked the front part of the body, do the same for the back and buttocks. If the hand-held mirror cannot reflect the area you may need to ask another person for help.

Examine both arms looking at all sides, including the armpit, palms of the hands, and underneath the fingernails. Then examine both thighs and legs, front and back. Examine your feet as well, including the soles of the feet, the toenails, and the area between the toes.

If you see any moles, areas of pigmentation (brown patches), or other lesions, remember where they are and what they look like. The most important clue to a melanoma is a skin lesion that has *changed* in some way. Once you start examining yourself regularly you will become familiar with your normal moles and skin lesions. That will make it easier to recognize one that has changed or when a new lesion appears. It is important to write down your findings and ask your doctor about any new or changing moles that concern you.

To help you remember exactly what your skin is like and where each mole is, it is useful to have a chart of the body to record the location of each mole. I have included body maps here, as well as in Appendix C, for your Early Detection Self-Exam. Make copies of the body maps and use them when you examine your skin to mark down the location of each mole as you go. Also write the date of each exam and keep the charts in a secure location. By comparing each month's charts to the last month you will be able to see at a glance if anything is new. Remember, if you find something of concern you should discuss it with your doctor.

When checking your skin during times of hormonal changes, such as during puberty, pregnancy, menopause, or when taking hormonal medications, be especially attentive. Hormones can change the appearance of some moles but without cause for alarm.

Remember that it is very common to have normal skin bumps, bruises, pimples, scabs, and other minor skin ailments that are not related to melanoma. These usually disappear within two to three weeks or have been there for years. Once you have a baseline, or preliminary, examination by a dermatologist, you will know which lumps and bumps are nothing and you can disregard them in your monthly exam.

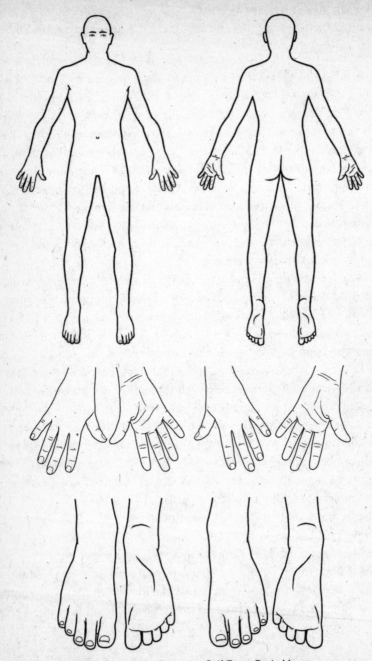

Figure 3-1. Early Detection Self-Exam Body Maps

Use the larger versions in the Appendix on pages 284–88 for photocopying.

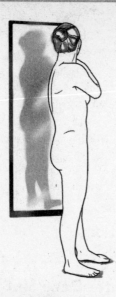

Figure 3-2. Standing in front of a full-length mirror, examine the skin from the top of the scalp to the bottom of the feet for moles or other lesions. Record and date them on the body map.

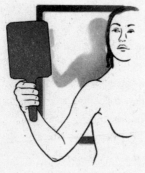

Figure 3-3. Use a hand-held mirror to completely inspect all areas of the body, especially on the back and buttocks, which may be difficult to see in front of the mirror. Alternatively, you can ask a close friend or relative to look at your back and tell you about any moles that may be difficult to see.

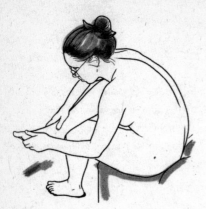

Figure 3-4. A complete skin examination includes the palms of the hands, soles of the feet, under the nails, and the area between the toes.

Columbia Melanoma Center Case Studies

Yvonne, a thirty-four-year-old woman, had had a mole on her left arm for many years. But over a period of about six weeks, she noticed that the mole had begun to change shape and was darker, prompting her to seek medical attention. Yvonne was otherwise healthy but enjoyed sunbathing and reported extensive exposure to sunlight during childhood and as an adult. She burned easily when in the sun but had no family history of melanoma. Her primary doctor had sent her to a dermatologist who performed a biopsy of the mole and found it was an early form of melanoma. Yvonne was referred to our center, where she underwent a successful removal of the melanoma. Fortunately, the melanoma was very thin and the risk of internal spread was practically zero. Yvonne came back to the clinic after her operation, wanting to know how she could prevent another melanoma from developing.

Yvonne represents a very common clinical situation: a melanoma that is identified at an early stage and completely controlled by a simple surgical procedure. Yvonne is correct, however, in worrying about developing a new melanoma since her risk is nearly nine hundred times that of the general population for such an occurrence. I told Yvonne that the best thing she could do was perform monthly skin examinations and use the body map to record any changes or new moles. The chance of a local recurrence—that is, the melanoma returning at the original site in her arm—is greatest during the first two years after removal. So I also advised her to see a dermatologist for skin screening every six months for the next two years and once a year thereafter. She was also advised to avoid the sun as much as possible. If she goes into the sun she should stay in shaded areas, wear protective clothing and ultraviolet protection sunglasses, and use sunscreen with an SPF of 45.

Ask Your Doctor

If you want to find out what you can do to prevent melanoma ask the following questions:

1. *How great is my risk for developing melanoma?* By considering your medical history, family history, and the biological features of any skin moles or tumors that have been removed, your doctor should be able to tell you if there is a significant risk for melanoma and then should be able to outline a plan of prevention that is best for you.

2. *Should I see a dermatologist?* Many dermatologists—but not all— provide professional screening for skin cancer and melanoma. Some dermatologists also take digital photographs to document any skin lesions or moles. If you are at moderate or high risk of melanoma then referral to such a dermatologist is indicated. Your primary physician should make this referral for you.

3. *How often should I see the dermatologist?* This depends on how significant your risk of melanoma is based on your medical history and family history. If the risk is low then you should see the dermatologist once a year. If the risk is moderate to high then a dermatology appointment may be necessary every six months. Only under rare circumstances, such as if you have a high-risk genetic disorder, would you need to see the dermatologist more frequently.

4. *Should I perform the Early Detection Self-Exam?* The Early Detection Self-Exam is easy to perform and costs nothing except your time, so

it is recommended for everyone and should be done on a regular basis. If your physician is not familiar with it you can ask to speak with a doctor or nurse who knows how to do it. Call the National Cancer Institute or the American Cancer Society for information (contact numbers and Web sites are in Appendix B on pages 280 and 282), or use the method I described. Although there is no proof that this will decrease the occurrence of melanoma, the exam may detect melanoma at a much earlier stage. Remember that you must call your doctor or dermatologist if you find anything unusual.

5. *What sunscreen product should I use?* Most physicians do not have a specific recommendation about a product. You can generally choose one that you like. I recommend an SPF of at least 30, especially if you will be out in the sun for a prolonged period of time. Reapply sunscreen after going in the water if it is not waterproof and every few hours regardless.

PART TWO

Diagnosing and Staging Melanoma

CHAPTER FOUR

How Do We Diagnose Melanoma?

I F YOU'VE READ this far, I'm betting you are taking precautions against sun exposure and doing regular skin self-examinations. The next step is to know what to do if, despite your diligence, you find a new mole or a mole that has changed. While you don't want to be unduly alarmist, such suspicious moles warrant an evaluation to rule out melanoma. The only way to be absolutely certain that a mole is actually a melanoma is for a trained pathologist to examine a sample under a microscope. The only way to obtain adequate tissue for the pathologist is through a minor procedure called a biopsy. One reason I always recommend a biopsy for suspicious looking moles is that even the best physicians find it difficult or nearly impossible to diagnose melanoma by just looking at a mole. A trained professional can tell what is really suspicious and what is not through visual inspection, but only biopsy can confirm a melanoma with 100 percent certainty. It is equally important that you see a doctor with specialized training in skin cancer and melanoma if you are concerned that a mole may be melanoma.

Signs and Symptoms of Melanoma

Every disease in medical practice can be described by symptoms that occur in patients. Symptoms are subjective complaints that patients experience, such as "my mole has become darker," or "my mole is hurting me now." Doctors are trained in understanding these symptoms in the context of specific diseases and also look for evidence of these diseases as manifested by certain characteristics that can be found on a physical examination of patients with the disease—so-called "signs" of the disease. A sign is an objective finding on physical examination. The diagnosis for many diseases can be made by an astute physician by comparing the symptoms a patient has with the signs observed on physical examination. This is why any change in your moles requires a visit to the doctor so he or she can hear about the symptoms and confirm the diagnosis by the signs found on an examination. Although the doctor may suspect melanoma, this must be confirmed by a biopsy of the suspicious mole.

While most melanomas occur on the skin (cutaneous melanoma), a small number of melanomas do not begin there and may be even more difficult to diagnose. I will discuss non-cutaneous melanoma in more detail in Chapter 9 because they behave so differently from cutaneous melanoma.

After the skin, the most frequent site for melanomas is in the eye (ocular melanoma). The other common site for melanoma outside the skin is in the mucous membranes around the mouth, nose, and sinus cavities of the face. These areas are protected by a specialized surface of mucous-producing cells that help facilitate body functions such as eating, speaking, and breathing. Melanocytes can be found in the layers of the mucous membranes, much like those throughout the surface of the skin, and so melanoma is *possible* but still unlikely: Only about 1 percent of all melanomas occur in the mucous membranes. Another part of the body that has a mucous membrane is around the anus. Anal melanoma may manifest as rectal pain or bleeding. In fact, melanomas that occur in the anal area are often mistaken for hemorrhoids. If you have hemorrhoids that do not heal with simple medical measures, have them evaluated by a doctor. (See Chapter 9 for more information.)

In 1 percent of all cases we cannot find the original or primary melanoma site. Most melanoma experts now agree that this situation likely occurs because the immune system has attacked and destroyed small melanomas in the skin without leaving behind any evidence on the skin or mucous membranes. The melanoma only becomes noticeable after spreading to the lymph nodes or internal organs.

Cutaneous Melanoma

Usually, the first symptom of cutaneous melanomas is the appearance of a new, pigmented lesion on an area of previously normal skin. As I have said, not all new moles are melanoma, and in fact most new, pigmented lesions are not melanoma. As we age, it is typical to acquire more lesions, some from sun exposure or just due to normal aging. It's easy for patients to mistake these for melanoma but they are not. Any new moles that are of concern should be pointed out to your doctor or dermatologist, who many times can reassure you that the lesion is not a melanoma. The trained professional can usually distinguish suspicious moles from benign skin lesions, but if there is any doubt a biopsy is indicated. Sometimes, melanoma will begin to grow from a mole that has been present for many years. Monthly self-examination is helpful because you will be so familiar with your "normal" moles, you will recognize when a normal mole begins to change. A changing mole almost always requires a biopsy. I have seen several patients whose dermatologists were not concerned about a mole, but when the patient told me that their mole had changed considerably I insisted on a biopsy. I almost always find a small melanoma in this situation which allows easy treatment. I think it is very important to listen to my patients.

Cutaneous melanomas can occur anywhere where there is skin. The chances for melanoma are about equally divided throughout the entire skin over the body. (See Table 4-1 for the frequency of melanoma at different parts of the body.) This democratic distribution means all sites, including the scalp under the hair and the space between the toes, should be carefully examined when you are concerned about a melanoma. In addition, a very small number, less than 1 percent of melanomas, may occur under the fingernails or toenails—a condition called subungual melanoma. Both patients and doctors often mistake a subungual melanoma for an infection or a hematoma (or blood clot). Although melanoma may occur under any nail, the thumb and great toe of the foot are the most frequently involved. If there is any abnormality of the nails that does not heal with simple treatment, such as antibiotics, a biopsy to exclude a melanoma is necessary.

Table 4-1. Locations of cutaneous melanomas

Location	Frequency
Head and neck	22%
Arms and hands	23%
Legs and feet	21%
Torso, front and back	34%
Under finger- and toenails	<1%

As a melanoma physician, I look for certain signs during a physical examination of the skin including the scalp, head, face, neck, arms, legs, front and back torso, and the nails, including in between each toe. Anyone can record the *presence* of moles—and you should—but the characteristic *appearance* of each mole is very significant to the trained eye. I teach my medical students the ABCDE signs of melanoma (see Table 4-2), which the American Cancer Society recommends, as a guide to determining which moles are most suspicious for melanoma. The A stands for asymmetry: Any mole that is not completely round and smooth is more likely to harbor a melanoma. The B stands for border irregularity and means that the edges of the mole are jagged or uneven. The C stands for color variegation; the color of the mole may change and contain differing shades of brown, black, red, or blue; sometimes there is no color and the melanoma can look white or tan colored. The D stands for diameter. Moles greater than five millimeters across, or about half the diameter of a penny, are more worrisome than smaller lesions. The E stands for enlargement and any mole that has grown is suspicious. I often tell my medical students that the most important factor is change, and we speak of the "E" in the ABDCE as not only "enlargement" but "evolution" since some melanomas will actually cause the mole to regress, or shrink. When my patient tells me that a mole has changed I pay close attention. I'd like to stress that any one sign alone is not *conclusive* for melanoma. A combination of these factors, however, makes me more concerned about melanoma.

Table 4-2. Signs of melanoma

Letter	Sign	Interpretation
A	Asymmetry	The mole is not smooth; the two sides appear different
B	Border irregularity	The edges of the mole are notched, blurred, or disrupted
C	Color variegation	Moles with variable color patterns
D	Diameter	Moles larger than 5 millimeters
E	Enlargement/Evolution	Moles that have grown or changed in any way

Signs and Symptoms of Advanced Melanoma

Melanoma that has spread to local lymph nodes usually occurs as a lump under the arms or in the groin, the two most common areas of lymph node involvement. Occasionally the lymph nodes in the neck and behind the knee or elbow can also contain melanoma. Typically, these lumps are not painful, and this lack of pain is often used to distinguish lymph nodes that have enlarged due to melanoma versus an infection. Painful lymph nodes often indicate an infection. Fortunately this is much more common than melanoma, and antibiotics may help. Any lumps in these areas that do not disappear in about two to three weeks with antibiotics are a serious symptom and you should see your doctor. Sometimes, if the nodes are very large, there can be swelling or discomfort in the arm or leg. On physical examination I feel the neck, under the arms, the groin, and behind the knees and elbows for any evidence of enlarged lymph nodes. I also note if there is any swelling or other abnormalities in the arms or legs.

When melanoma spreads to internal organs the symptoms relate to the organ involved. For example, patients often complain of chest pain, shortness of breath, or coughing spells when melanoma spreads to the lungs. When a melanoma spreads to the liver it is not uncommon to experience right-sided abdominal pain, difficulty eating and digesting food, and perhaps jaundice. If melanoma spreads into the brain, patients may experience severe headaches, numbness and weakness of the arms or legs, and, rarely, seizures. The most common complaint though is a general feeling of fatigue, or extreme tiredness. This is often accompanied by poor appetite and weight loss. These symptoms are common for many, many medical and psychiatric illnesses and so they have to be evaluated by a physician before making any definite conclusions. Nonetheless, these symptoms are very serious and a full physical examination and medical testing should be done to make sure that melanoma is not the culprit. I discuss this in more detail in Chapter 8.

Making the Diagnosis: Biopsy

Once I've applied the ABCDE criteria, and I think a lesion likely benign and not a melanoma, then I still recommend careful observation. I tell patients to keep watching it and return if there are any further changes. On the other hand, if I'm concerned enough about the mole and want to diagnose it, I will recommend a biopsy, or removal of some, or all, of the lesion with microscopic evaluation of the cells. When melanoma is a possibility it is essential to obtain a piece of intact skin for evaluation. Many benign skin conditions can be safely and easily treated with a shaving (shave biopsy), freezing (cryotherapy), or laser (laser therapy) technique. These methods destroy the lesion completely and do not provide sufficient material for a pathologist to examine under the microscope. Therefore, if there is any concern about melanoma, a regular biopsy should be done. In general, biopsy of the skin is a minor procedure that can be conducted in the doctor's office. One of several acceptable methods is chosen, depending on the size of the mole and the expertise of the doctor performing the procedure.

If the mole is very small, a *punch biopsy* can be done. A small device, with a plastic handle and a circular metal core similar to a paper hole puncher, "punches" out an anesthetized piece of skin over the mole. Skin punches are typically three- or four-millimeter-diameter pieces of cone-shaped skin; often a single stitch or a piece of adhesive tape can be used to close the wound. The site usually heals completely in about a week or two. The punch removes enough skin for the pathologist to make a detailed examination of the mole.

If the lesion is larger than about four millimeters it may be necessary to take a larger biopsy. An *excisional biopsy* is a surgical technique that uses a scalpel and attempts to remove the entire lesion. Done with a local anesthetic, it can be performed in an office setting as well by a dermatologist with skill in the technique or by a surgeon. When the mole is fairly small the excisional biopsy can remove the entire lesion. Excisional biopsy usually requires a few stitches and takes a few more days to heal. When I perform an excisional biopsy I typically use dissolving stitches, which results in excellent healing, less scar formation, and no need for removing stitches later.

If the mole is extremely large then I may opt to remove only a small piece for evaluation before attempting definitive treatment. Either a punch biopsy or a surgical approach to take a portion of the lesion (called an *incisional biopsy*) may be used. In this case the punch biopsy or incision is taken from the most suspicious looking area of the mole, which allows for the best chance for obtaining tissue for the pathologist to examine and make a diagnosis.

A biopsy is considered a minor procedure and the risks are very small. But all procedures have some degree of risk. The risks of a biopsy by a trained dermatologist or surgeon are very low. The most common risks of a biopsy are bleeding and infection. Bleeding may be more of a problem if you are taking blood thinning medication or if you have a blood clotting disorder. Do tell your doctor if you are taking aspirin, which can thin the blood, or any other medication. Then she or he can deal with any excess bleeding or have you stop taking your medication for a few days before the biopsy. Infection is so uncommon that I do not usually take any extra precautions. If you have an illness that may increase the chances of an infection then you can take antibiotics before the biopsy. There is also a small risk of having an allergic reaction to the local anesthetic, so tell your doctor if you have any known allergies.

If the biopsy leaves an open area of the skin, stitches or adhesive tapes can easily close it. Many surgeons now use dissolvable stitches that dissolve once the skin is healed, about six weeks later. If the biopsy is located in an area that is subjected to extra stress, like the sole of the foot, stronger stitches may be used. In this case the stitches may need to be removed five to seven days after the biopsy. Your doctor should be able to explain exactly which procedure he or she will use.

I want to be quite clear that a biopsy is used as a diagnostic tool. *The biopsy does not represent adequate treatment for melanoma.* It is only done to determine if the mole is a melanoma and to provide additional information about the melanoma, which I will discuss later. For now, please realize how essential it is to return to your doctor after a biopsy to hear your diagnosis and determine what next steps are needed for treatment. Improperly treated melanoma can return to the same site if not completely removed.

The biopsy procedure is simple and the biopsy site usually heals quickly. The segment of skin with the suspicious mole is sent to the pathologist, an expert physician trained in the diagnosis of disease by microscopic evaluation. In some cases, skin lesions are reviewed by a dermatopathologist, a pathologist with additional training in skin diseases. The pathologist will examine the skin sample under a microscope after staining the cells with special dyes that highlight features of the exposed cells, an examination critical to the diagnosis of melanoma. The pathologist will look for certain features, such as the general appearance of the melanocytes, their location, their contact with other melanocytes, and the appearance of the cell's nucleus (the center of the cell that contains the chromosomes). These general features are used to distinguish normal melanocytes from melanoma cells. In addition, there are several special stains that can be used to determine the presence of proteins that are found only on melanoma cells. The results of the pathologist's examination, including any special stains used, is detailed in a document called the "pathology report," and this report is sent to your doctor following a biopsy. If a melanoma is present, certain features of it determine the outcome (or prognosis) of the disease and may help determine what treatment options will be helpful. This information is how we stage or categorize melanoma, which I will discuss in detail in the next chapter. Keep in mind that this information is only possible by a biopsy and careful review of the specimen by a trained pathologist.

One other technique sometimes used to diagnose melanoma is *fine needle aspiration*, in which a small needle is inserted into a skin lesion or tumor several times. The tissue obtained is immediately placed on a glass slide under the microscope for a trained pathologist, called a cytopathologist or cytologist, to examine. The cytologist is an expert at identifying tumors with only a small number of cells obtained by a needle, rather than looking at an entire area of skin. Like pathologists, the cytologist can often use special stains to increase the chances of finding melanoma cells. In our center the cytologist actually comes to the clinic with a microscope to examine the aspirate immediately. If there are insufficient cells we can repeat the procedure until a diagnosis is made.

Although fine needle aspiration is helpful for identifying melanoma, there are several caveats. First, it is always possible that the sample removed may miss the real tumor, so a negative result has to be interpreted cautiously. Second, this technique can find melanoma cells but does not give any information about the depth of the melanoma or whether the melanoma is ulcerated. A biopsy must be done to determine these features. Fine needle aspiration, however, is very useful for determining if melanoma has spread to lymph nodes or other sites where a lump can be easily felt by the physician.

Histologic Types of Melanoma

If a melanoma is identified in the biopsy specimen, your doctor will get additional information by careful evaluation of the cells. The most important feature is the depth of the melanoma. We know that the behavior of melanoma is closely related to how deep the melanoma has grown into the skin. A very thin melanoma is easily cured and has little likelihood of spreading anywhere. A deep melanoma, however, is much more serious and has a higher chance of breaking off from the skin and spreading to other sites in the body. Most pathologists will report a depth for every melanoma that they examine. This measurement is among the most significant factors for making medical decisions.

The other thing that can be determined on microscopic review of melanoma specimens is the presence of skin ulceration over the area of the melanoma. As you know, the skin is composed of specialized cells that provide a barrier against the outside environment. An ulcer of the skin occurs when the cells of the skin are destroyed or missing and this may happen over areas where melanomas are growing. This particular feature is now linked to the behavior of melanomas since those with areas of ulceration tend to be more aggressive. We cannot usually detect ulceration with our eyes, so pathologists need to look for this when they examine the skin under the microscope.

Today we know that the depth of the melanoma and the presence of ulceration are the two most common findings the pathologist describes, but only recently have they been included in the official pathology report. Before, pathologists often described a number of different histologic, or cell subtypes of melanoma. Most experts now believe that these categories are not that important since the depth and ulceration are the only two things that determine the behavior of melanoma. I want to describe subtypes, however, since they are often mentioned by pathologists and may have some clinical importance in a few cases.

Superficial Spreading Melanoma

The superficial spreading melanoma is the most common type and accounts for 60–70 percent of all melanoma cases. The name refers to the ability of the melanoma cells to spread across the superficial layers of the skin before spreading into the deeper parts of the skin. Although this sounds ominous, the early superficial spreading process may take many years. These melanomas often start in a previously normal mole and as the mole enlarges, the patient notices it. These types of melanoma are typically flat or barely raised and often contain various shades of brown or black. Although superficial spreading melanoma can occur anywhere, it's most common on the legs in women and the torso in men, and mostly in younger and middle-aged adults.

Nodular Melanoma

This form occurs in 15–30 percent of patients with melanoma and often appears as a dark black-blue or bluish-red solid nodule of almost any size. In some cases there is no pigment and the nodule may be flesh-colored or white in appearance. These types of melanoma often occur in previously normal areas of skin rather than from an existing mole. They grow deeper early on and can spread more quickly than superficial spreading melanomas. Although experts once thought that these melanomas had a worse prognosis, the current thinking is that superficial spreading and nodular melanomas of the same depth will behave in the same manner, but we are more likely to find nodular melanomas at a deeper depth at the time of diagnosis. Because these melanomas are often deep when they are diagnosed, the prognosis is generally worse than that for superficial spreading melanomas. For unknown reasons, nodular melanoma is more common in men and tends to occur on the head and neck or torso regions. Nodular melanoma is also more common in a slightly older population.

Lentigo Maligna Melanoma

The lentigo maligna melanoma, which accounts for approximately 5 percent of melanoma lesions, occurs on the face, and sometimes the back of the hands. They appear as flat brown shaded lesions and can be large enough to cover the entire cheek. There are usually associated areas of sun-damaged skin near these melanomas. The lentigo maligna melanoma is more common in women and occurs in older patients. These melanomas are less likely than the others to spread and so they have a generally good prognosis.

Acral Lentiginous Melanoma

Although these melanomas are not common—less than 5 percent of all melanomas—almost 70 percent of the melanomas that affect African Americans and 50 percent of Asians are acral lentiginous. Usually located on the soles of the feet, and sometimes on the palms of the hands, acral lentiginous melanoma is often not diagnosed until an advanced stage. Therefore, the outcome may be poor. The melanoma appears as a brown, black, tan, or mixed-color lesion with very irregular borders and various sizes. (Note: Not all melanomas on these sites are acral lentiginous.)

Subungual Melanoma

These melanomas make up 1–3 percent of all melanomas and occur under a fingernail or toenail, most commonly in the thumb or great toe. Subungual melanomas are often mistaken for something else, most commonly a hematoma (blood collection) following traumatic injury of the finger or toe. Occasionally the lesions may be mistaken for a fungal infection of the nail. These melanomas often appear as a blackened area on the side or base of the nail and are usually irregular and larger than three millimeters. Subungual melanomas tend to occur in patients over fifty years old, although this is not always the case. They also occur more frequently in people of African American, Asian, and Native American descent. Nail discoloration or masses that do not heal within four to six weeks should prompt removal of the nail and a biopsy.

Desmoplastic Melanoma

A rare form that has only been recognized as a distinct entity since the early 1970s, desmoplastic melanoma typically has areas of fibrotic, or inflammatory, tissue surrounding the melanoma cells. The desmoplastic melanoma is often very aggressive and tends to come back even after surgical removal. Therefore, patients with desmoplastic melanoma need to be monitored closely. The small number of cases and the relatively recent identification of desmoplastic melanoma means there is little long-term data available on the natural history of this type of melanoma. If you have desmoplastic melanoma you need to be followed even more closely by a melanoma expert.

A Note on Size

In reading about these different subtypes, you may have concluded that the size of the melanoma on the skin is not an important distinguishing feature. It is generally true that the size of the melanoma on the skin has little impact on the outcome of treatment for melanoma. I would like to clarify this point, however. When melanomas begin in the skin they first start to grow in the superficial layers of the skin. This growth can be identified as an increase in the size or appearance of a mole or the start of a new mole. The more a mole grows the more likely it is to be a melanoma. Therefore, size helps us to identify melanoma in the early stages. Those moles that are bigger than five millimeters, or about half the diameter of a penny, are more likely to have melanoma than small moles. After the melanoma grows along the superficial layers of the skin, the cells may start to grow deeper into the skin where they can cause problems, including the ability to spread as they encounter the lymphatic system. Again, the total diameter of the melanoma on the surface of the skin is less important than the depth of the melanoma in the deeper layers of the skin.

The Doctors Who Deal with Melanoma

When confronted with a potentially serious illness like melanoma, it is imperative to gather information, ask your doctors questions, and make sure that you feel comfortable with the medical decisions and procedures you are considering. There is little doubt that making the diagnosis as early as possible is beneficial for living with melanoma. Likewise, making certain that you have the right type of treatment as soon as possible may improve your chances of cure and living a long life. This is your health and you deserve to have the best possible care. There is no one doctor who deals with all aspects of melanoma and so it is important that you understand whom to see and what each specialist has to offer. Here is a brief rundown of the many types of doctors that you might see, hear about, or need to ask for referral to if you are dealing with melanoma or think you might have melanoma.

The particular type of doctor you should see depends in part on the stage of melanoma, and in part on who is available in your area and through your insurance plan. I present the most common types of physicians in the order you are likely to encounter them. You should eventually see an expert in this disease since your chance of a successful outcome and the ability to live with melanoma depends on receiving the best possible care. In my experience, most health care insurance companies are willing to provide a referral to a melanoma specialist since the cost of definitive care early on is always less than if the wrong treatments are used.

Primary Care Physician

Your primary physician takes responsibility for your overall health and well-being. Usually trained in internal medicine or family practice, primary care physicians for children and adolescents may be pediatricians. Similarly, some women see an obstetrician-gynecologist for their primary health care. These physicians have your general medical history and may be familiar with your family and personal medical history. They often participate in screening programs; they may or may not be familiar with skin cancer and skin cancer prevention techniques. They most likely will not be experts in melanoma and will not be able to perform a biopsy. Do feel free to ask your primary care physician about his or her experience with melanoma. You have the right to a referral to another type of doctor for evaluation, diagnosis, and treatment if there is any question.

Dermatologist

A physician with advanced training in diseases of the skin, including skin cancer and melanoma, this is often the doctor who has the most experience in identifying skin cancers and melanomas by visual inspection. Some dermatologists specialize in skin cancer screening and can provide you with both a professional examination and information on how to prevent melanoma. Most dermatologists are also skilled at performing small biopsy procedures, including punch biopsies. Some dermatologists with an interest in surgery may also be able to perform minor surgical operations. Many dermatologists also offer digital photography of the skin as a way to document skin lesions. Taking the photographs of the same area on a regular basis helps them to identify changes in particular skin lesions. Called mole mapping, this process has not been widely adopted yet and although digital photography has not been proven as a method for enhancing melanoma prevention, it offers some people peace of mind.

Surgical Oncologist

A general surgeon with specialized training in the surgical treatment of cancer is called a surgical oncologist. Surgery is the main treatment for early-stage and some late-stage melanomas and the surgical oncologist is usually called in to perform these procedures. These surgeons are usually well versed in the proper treatment for all stages of melanoma and can perform both simple biopsy procedures and complex operations for melanoma. The surgical oncologist who specializes in melanoma is familiar with all aspects of melanoma, although some surgical oncologists specialize in only certain tumors. Your primary care physician may refer you directly to the surgeon instead of a dermatologist for management. A general surgeon, as opposed to a surgical oncologist, also has the necessary skills for performing a biopsy and simple surgical procedures but may not be an expert in the management of melanoma. Ask your surgeon about his or her experience with melanoma and whether he has a colleague with more skill in taking care of melanoma patients.

Plastic Surgeon

With specialized training in cosmetic and reconstructive procedures, the plastic surgeon repairs, remodels, or restores body parts, including the skin. Some plastic surgeons are able to perform biopsies and even treatment procedures for melanoma. They are often called in to help when the melanoma is located on a particularly difficult part of the body, such as the nose or ear, or other areas where removing large pieces of skin will leave a large defect. In general, though, most plastic surgeons are not trained in the management of cancer and will usually coordinate care of patients with other physicians who have this experience. For example, I often call on our plastic surgeons to help when I remove a large melanoma from the face. This allows me to make certain that the entire melanoma is removed, and the plastic surgeon can help close the wound with the least scarring possible.

Pathologist

A physician with expert training in the diagnosis of disease through the examination of tissues and cells, the pathologist is an essential member of the team and is responsible for processing biopsy and tissue specimens and making the diagnosis. The pathologist may perform special stains on the tumor specimen and report this information to the dermatologist or surgeon. Pathologists with advanced training in diseases of the skin are called dermatopathologists. If there is any concern about the interpretation of a specimen it should be sent to an expert dermatopathologist for confirmation, as this is among the most important pieces of information needed to plan treatment.

Radiologist

A radiologist specializes in the use of X-rays for diagnostic purposes. If necessary, the radiologist may be called on to take X-rays or a CAT scan, write up a report on the results, and send them directly to the physician ordering the scan. In addition, an interventional radiologist may apply therapeutic interventions for patients using X-ray guidance to find small tumors, a relatively new experimental approach to the treatment of cancer. An interventional radiologist locates melanomas deep inside internal organs by X-ray imaging methods and then directs some type of drug to the precise location. This approach allows a way to get high doses of chemotherapy, vaccines, and other drugs close to a melanoma. Another strategy has been to use the local approach to cut off the blood vessels and essentially "starve" the melanoma. More research with these techniques is needed, but the interventional radiologist is starting to play a larger role in the management of complicated melanomas.

Medical Oncologist

A physician with advanced training in the treatment of cancer and related diseases, the medical oncologist usually has internal medicine training and is an expert in the administration of chemotherapy. It is the medical oncologist that usually coordinates the care of patients with advanced cancers, including melanoma. However, in the early stages of cancers such as melanoma, the dermatologist or surgical oncologist may be the coordinating physician.

Radiation Oncologist

The radiation oncologist is a specialist in the use of radiation for the treatment of cancer, and is often called upon for controlling melanoma that has spread to certain locations, such as the bones or brain.

IN ADDITION TO these physicians, additional specialists may be needed for unique circumstances. For example, if a melanoma is located in the head or neck region, an otorhinolaryngologist, or "ear, nose, and throat" doctor may be called upon. If melanoma spreads to the lungs a pulmonologist, an expert in diseases of the lungs, may be helpful. Likewise, if melanoma occurs in the brain or spinal cord, a neurosurgeon will likely be necessary if surgical removal is possible.

There are so many potential experts who could be involved, you may feel overwhelmed or confused. I suggest my patients choose one physician with whom they have a good, trusting relationship to act as their "main" physician. This is both comforting for the patient and more efficient for the health care providers, as many tests need to be ordered and reviewed, and referrals may need to be made to a wide range of doctors and services. Another very important point in choosing your main doctor is time. Every day you wait slowly shuts your window of opportunity in terms of receiving treatment before your disease has advanced.

I realize people fear hurting their doctors' feelings, but in truth you are doing them a favor. When a general physician or surgeon refers a patient to me, I am always happy to keep them informed. Remember you are a consumer of your health care and your own best advocate. If you were shopping for a refrigerator, you wouldn't hesitate to go to the store you liked the best.

The physician you choose as your coordinating doctor may depend on the stage of disease. A dermatologist or surgical oncologist is usually best for early stage melanoma. A medical oncologist or surgical oncologist is often better for late stage melanoma. Especially with a disease like melanoma, in which no one standardized treatment exists, it's crucial to find the specialist with the most up to date and expert knowledge of both standard and experimental treatment. In the next few chapters I will point out which type of physician is best for specific procedures.

Columbia Melanoma Center Case Studies

Frederick, a seventy-two-year-old man, came to my office when a mole he had had on his right shoulder for many years began to grow and change shape. He also thought that the mole had become somewhat darker during the last month. There was no history of melanoma in any of his family, as far as he knew. He did tell me that he occasionally developed severe sunburns when he was out in the sun. When I examined him I found a six millimeter brownish black mole with an irregular edge on his right shoulder. There were no other abnormalities on his examination, and he had no other medical problems.

Frederick agreed to let me perform a small punch biopsy in the office.

One week later, the pathology report confirmed the diagnosis of melanoma. Frederick underwent surgery to remove the entire area of the melanoma, including a margin of the healthy skin surrounding it. He healed quickly and I told him to avoid excessive sun exposure and return for regular examinations of the skin every twelve months. I have now known Frederick for many years and consider him cured of his melanoma.

Ask Your Doctor

If you have a suspicious mole and are concerned about melanoma, ask the following questions:

1. *Do you recommend that I have a biopsy?* There is no other definitive way to be certain that a mole is melanoma. If the mole is small enough, a punch biopsy or a surgical biopsy may remove it entirely. Ask your doctor about their experience doing this procedure and have them explain how they will do it and when they will examine you again. Also make sure that the specimen is sent to an experienced pathologist for review and ask to hear about the pathology report when it is ready, typically in about five to seven days. If your doctor does not recommend a biopsy, ask what he thinks the diagnosis is, his plans for observing the mole, and what will be done if the mole does not get better. You may need to seek another doctor if you remain concerned about a mole that continues to grow or change for more than four to six weeks.

2. *Do you perform mole mapping or use some type of photography to document my skin lesions?* Some dermatologists have a system for mole mapping, which may include digital photographs of your skin. This is an especially useful way to examine moles at different times, but has not yet been validated and cannot substitute for an examination by a physician trained in recognizing melanoma and other skin disorders. Once a suspicious mole is identified, your doctor should have a plan for carefully following the mole. This may include regular skin examinations by a dermatologist, instruction on how to perform self-examination of the skin (which is also explained

in Chapter 3), and education on how you can prevent melanoma (also discussed in Chapter 3).

3. *What is your experience in the diagnosis and treatment of melanoma?* You have every right to know about your doctor's experience with specific diseases and topics. Most reliable doctors do not mind these questions and are usually willing to refer you to their colleagues with appropriate expertise. I am often asked how many patients I treat with melanoma or how many years I have been involved with melanoma treatment. My response is always positive since I know anyone who asks this is intelligent and is asking me the right kind of questions! It is better to be sure that you are getting the best possible care than to worry about offending your doctor.

4. *What type of biopsy do you recommend? Why?* Most melanoma experts prefer to perform a punch biopsy whenever possible. This biopsy allows enough tissue to be removed for the pathologist to examine and results in minimal disruption of the skin. Healing is usually quite rapid after a punch biopsy and only occasionally requires a stitch to close. If the mole is larger than four millimeters, an excisional biopsy can usually be done in an office setting. This type of biopsy usually heals quickly as well but may require stitches to close the skin. An incisional biopsy may be performed when the mole is very large or in an unusual location. This type of biopsy removes only a portion of the mole for examination, so the pathologist may not be able to make a final diagnosis. Whatever the procedure, you should understand that the biopsy does not represent treatment. The treatment is based on the results of the biopsy.

5. *What are the risks of the biopsy?* The main risks are bleeding, infection, allergic reactions, and recurrence of the melanoma. These are usually minimal but may be more serious in people with medical illnesses that affect the blood clotting system and immune system, or those taking certain medications that affect these systems. You should tell your doctor about any medical problems, medications, or allergies before a biopsy or any surgical procedure.

6. *When do I need to come back?* I see my biopsy patients one week later so that I can make sure they are healing and so we can discuss the pathology report. Occasionally we need to send the pathology specimen for special stains and it may take longer to have a final report with the diagnosis. Depending on how the biopsy was performed, your medical condition, and the pathology review process, you may be asked to come back sooner or later than one week, but you should be told in advance.

7. *Do you have a board certified dermatopathologist to review the biopsy sample?* This question is rarely asked but is among the most important pieces of information to obtain. Although it is not essential that the biopsy specimen be reviewed by a dermatopathologist, you should ask your doctor about the report, the level of certainty for the pathologist reviewing the specimen, and whether your doctor is comfortable with the diagnosis. If there is any hesitation or concern you may want to ask that the specimen be sent to another dermatopathologist with expertise in melanoma. Be patient since the diagnosis can sometimes be very difficult and even experts may disagree. It will be worth the wait to gather a consensus of opinions so that you can have the most appropriate treatment.

8. *What is the diagnosis?* The most important question to ask when the pathology report is reviewed: Is the mole a melanoma? If not, what is it?

9. *If this is not melanoma, what additional studies or further follow-up care do I need?* If the pathologist believes the mole is not melanoma then ask your doctor about treatment and long-term follow-up depending on the diagnosis. For most benign moles no further treatment will be necessary. The presence of many moles itself may increase the risk of melanoma, so self-examination of the skin and other measures to protect against sun exposure are good ideas.

10. *Whom do you recommend if I need further surgery?* If melanoma is confirmed a surgical procedure is almost always indicated, and you may need to be referred to a surgical oncologist or dermatologic surgeon who specializes in surgery for melanoma. The doctor

performing surgery may or may not be the one performing the biopsy. Ask the doctor explaining the biopsy results about their experience in surgical treatment and whom they would recommend for further therapy. The extent of surgery depends on features of the melanoma—information provided by staging—and determines the type of doctor needed for treatment. If the melanoma is located on the face you may need to see a plastic surgeon or a head and neck surgeon.

CHAPTER FIVE

The Melanoma Staging System

I N THE CLASSIC Hollywood or television scene depicting a person receiving the results of a positive biopsy or pathology report the patient asks, "Doctor . . . how long have I got?" I've heard this question countless times in my office. If the patient is reluctant to ask, invariably a family member wants to know the answer. Of course, no doctor can predict the future with any guarantee, no matter how much information and experience he has. But there is a scientific method for assessing how widespread the disease is in an individual. Armed with that information, we can at least provide anxious patients and their families with a general prognosis.

Staging is the process that doctors who specialize in cancer—the oncologists—use to define how advanced the cancer is at the time of diagnosis. The American Joint Committee on Cancer, or AJCC, has developed a system for cancer staging that is used by physicians and other health care professionals throughout the world. Every type of cancer has been assigned its own staging system. Accurate classification—or staging—permits appropriate treatment for a given stage of disease, allows doctors to better evaluate results of studies for different types of cancer, and provides a way to compare worldwide statistics about cancer and various treatments.

Since cancer research is going on all the time and new information becomes available regularly, melanoma staging must adapt to accommodate new information. Whenever especially important findings occur, an international committee is convened to review the current staging system and recommend changes. The AJCC has been very active in melanoma staging recently due to a surge of new knowledge. The staging system was updated in 1997 and then again in 2001, based on a more careful review of large numbers of patient medical records and an evaluation of the medical literature related to melanoma clinical studies.

The physicians and scientific researchers use this new information to compare patients with similar stages of disease and determine the best treatment options for each stage. Staging also means physicians can make a prognosis—in other words, how long a patient may have to live. All cancers need to be staged before doctors can tell you your prognosis or recommend an appropriate treatment.

Besides helping in the present, staging is a boon to the future of cancer treatment: staging permits scientists to study new treatments. When new drugs are tested it is important that they are given to patients with a similar stage of disease; drugs may be useful when the amount of disease is limited and less useful when it is widespread. By staging the disease, physicians and scientists can conduct studies across the world and compare the results because all the patients have a similar degree of cancer.

The staging of cancer is based on general principles that are relevant to all types of cancer. Three characteristics describe the outcome for most cancers, including melanoma. If you have been diagnosed with melanoma you will be given a TNM staging. In this system the "T" stands for "tumor" (or the primary cancer), the "N" stands for "lymph nodes," and the "M" stands for "metastasis." (The "TNM" staging system should not be confused with the simplified numerical staging most patients are familiar with and which I'll also explain below.) Your treatment depends entirely on your TNM staging, a system used by physicians all over the world to describe individual cancer patients.

1. T—THE TUMOR, OR PRIMARY CANCER

The first characteristic is the nature of the primary cancer itself.

The primary, or original, cancer is the first cancer to be detected and is found in the organ causing the cancer. In the case of melanoma, the cancer usually starts in the skin and so the primary cancer is found on the skin. Likewise, a primary lung cancer occurs in the lung and a primary breast cancer occurs in the breast, and so on. While this is generally true, melanoma is quite unpredictable and may not behave like other tumors. In about five percent of cases, no primary or original tumor is found. Instead, the melanoma is detected in the lymph nodes or internal organs, in which case, we stage according to the other criteria listed below.

For most cancers though, it is *the size of the primary cancer* that determines the outcome and how well patients will respond to treatment. The size is usually reported as the single largest dimension of measurement. In the case of breast cancer, for example, if the cancer is less than five centimeters the prognosis is better than for those cancers that are larger than five centimeters. For melanoma, however, the actual size of the tumor is not that important. The most significant feature of the primary melanoma is how thick it is, which explains why it is so important to have a biopsy of intact skin for the pathologist to measure the melanoma's thickness.

2. N—THE LYMPH NODES

The second characteristic that determines the stage of a cancer is whether or not the primary cancer *has spread to the nearby lymph nodes*. Lymph nodes are part of the immune system and serve as sites for generating an immune response. Every person typically has hundreds to thousands of lymph nodes throughout the body. Interestingly, many cancers often spread to the closest lymph nodes before spreading anywhere else. Therefore, for staging purposes, we always evaluate the lymph nodes closest to a cancer. In the case of internal cancers these lymph nodes are often removed at the time of surgery for the primary cancer. Dealing with the adjacent lymph nodes in melanoma can be tricky because they may be found in so many different places, depending on where the primary melanoma is located. The presence of melanoma in lymph nodes is more serious than if the primary melanoma has not spread at all, and this is true for all types of cancer. Another important prognostic tool is the number of lymph nodes that contain melanoma cells. The greater the number of lymph nodes that contain melanoma, the worse the prognosis becomes.

3. M—METASTASIS

The third factor in staging is the *presence of cancer in other organs of the body* far away from the primary cancer or lymph nodes. This process is called metastasis and for almost all cancers is a sign of a very poor prognosis. Unfortunately, melanoma can spread to almost any other organ in the body. Recently, it has become clear that the prognosis may depend on which organs are involved with melanoma. In its recent staging review, the AJCC noted that when melanoma spread to the skin or areas just below the skin including lymph nodes the survival rate was much better than when the melanoma had spread to the lungs. Surprisingly, patients with melanoma that had spread to the lungs did better and lived longer than patients whose melanoma had spread to any other internal organ.

We can predict prognosis based on whether the melanoma is found only in the skin, or has also spread to the lymph nodes or internal organs. Each case is individual and may respond differently. In general, over 80 percent of patients with melanoma confined to the skin will survive for at least five years (more than 90 percent if the melanoma is thin). Once the melanoma has spread to the lymph nodes, 50 percent of patients will be alive five years later. The most sobering news is that less than 10 percent of patients with melanoma that has spread to the internal organs will survive five years or more. These numbers may seem scary but I hope they help you to understand why it is so important to

learn about melanoma and diagnose it at an early stage. In giving my patients a prognosis, I stress that melanoma can be unpredictable and I
have many, many patients who are able to beat the odds and live a long
life even after melanoma has spread.

TNM Staging

Now I'll guide you through the staging process step by step, beginning with what the TNM code means and then what to expect from the
various tests involved to determine your TNM designation.

T Staging

When staging melanoma, instead of looking at the size of a tumor
alone, we measure its thickness or depth in the skin: The deeper the tumor the higher the T stage. As long as the melanoma is thin enough to
remain in the epidermis there is no chance of it spreading anywhere else
in the body. Once the melanoma begins to grow into the dermis—the
layer below the epidermis—the spread of melanoma is possible. The actual probability of spread is directly related to the thickness or depth of
the melanoma within the dermis. That is because melanoma travels
through the lymphatic channels, which are located in the deeper layers
of the dermis. If melanoma enters these channels the cells can travel
to the lymph nodes, and from there can enter into the general circulation toward the rest of the body. Table 5-1 defines the T stages for
melanoma. If the melanoma does not grow into the dermis, it is a T0.
A T1 melanoma is less than one millimeter thick, a T2 melanoma is
one–two millimeters thick, and so on. Once the melanoma is thicker
than four millimeters the chance of spread is very high.

The presence of ulceration is also part of the T stage designation. An
ulcer occurs when the skin over the melanoma becomes destroyed.
Sometimes this leads to mild bleeding at the melanoma site, making ulceration readily apparent. In other cases, although the skin is destroyed,

the ulceration cannot be detected by the naked eye but requires the expert opinion of the pathologist looking under a microscope. If ulceration is present, the letter "B" is added to the T stage; if there is no ulceration, then the T stage includes a letter "A." A melanoma that is two millimeters thick and has no signs of ulceration would be called a stage T2A. A melanoma that is three millimeters thick with ulceration would be called stage T3B.

Table 5-1. The T staging for melanoma

T0	Melanoma remains above the epidermis (in situ)	
T1	Less than 1.0 millimeters thick (into the dermis)	
T2	1–2 millimeters thick	A means no ulceration; B means ulceration
T3	2–4 millimeters thick	
T4	Greater than 4 millimeters thick	

N Staging

Occasionally a doctor can feel enlarged lymph nodes under the surface of the skin by manual examination alone, but small lymph nodes are usually not detectable. Therefore, to determine the N stage definitively, a pathologist examines the lymph nodes following their removal during surgery. If the primary melanoma is very thin, generally less than one millimeter, there is little chance of spread to the lymph nodes, so we usually do not remove them. However, when the melanoma is deeper than one millimeter, it is imperative to evaluate the nearby lymph nodes.

Which lymph nodes are removed for N staging depends on where the primary melanoma is located. In general, the closer the melanoma is to a site, the more likely that the melanoma will spread to that area. For melanomas in the head and neck the involved lymph nodes are usually found in the neck region. For melanomas on the arms the major lymph nodes are located in the armpit. For melanomas on the legs the local lymph nodes are usually in the groin, although for lower leg melanomas sometimes the lymph nodes behind the knee are involved. The local lymph nodes for the chest, abdomen, and back represent a real problem since melanoma can spread to either the armpits or the groin. I always manually examine the surface of these sites just to be sure.

You can see in Table 5-2 that the N stage depends on how many lymph nodes contain melanoma. If melanoma has not spread to the nearby lymph nodes the N stage is called N0. Based on following a large group of melanoma patients, we can safely assume that the more lymph nodes involved the worse the outcome. Once four lymph nodes are involved, however, the presence of more lymph nodes does not make the prognosis any worse.

Another significant factor is whether the melanoma is so small it is only detectable by careful microscopic examination after surgical removal of the lymph node. In the case of detection by microscope alone an "A" is added to the N staging; melanoma in two lymph nodes detected only after microscopic examination would be called N2A. If the lymph nodes can be detected by physical examination and the pathologist confirms melanoma after surgery, then a "B" designation is added, so one large lymph node confirmed by biopsy is called N1B.

A third situation may occur only with melanoma is in an arm or leg. The melanoma cells may start to spread but before reaching the lymph nodes they get "stuck" in the lymphatic vessels and begin to grow. When we see multiple small cancer growths just below the skin and scattered throughout the arm or leg, we add to the N stage a "C" designation, indicating melanoma cells are en route to the lymph nodes. An NC has a worse prognosis than if the melanoma is only found in the lymph nodes.

Table 5-2. The N staging for melanoma

N0	No lymph nodes contain melanoma	
N1	Melanoma in one lymph node	A: melanoma detectable only on microscopic examination B: melanoma also felt on physical examination C: in-transit melanoma
N2	Melanoma in 2–3 lymph nodes	
N3	Melanoma in 4 or more lymph nodes	

The M Staging

The outcome for patients with metastatic spread depends on the location in the body where the melanoma has spread. This information is conveyed in the M staging system. If no metastases are present then we state that the melanoma has an M0 stage. If metastases are present then the M stage is M1. Table 5-3 shows that when the melanoma is found only in the skin and soft tissues—located at other areas than the primary cancer—it is called M1A disease. If the melanoma spreads to the lungs, it is M1B melanoma. When the melanoma spreads to any other part of the body it is called M1C melanoma.

Another factor that appears to influence the outcome for patients with metastatic melanoma is an elevated lactate dehydrogenase (or LDH) marker in the blood. If a blood test reveals LDH is elevated, patients have an M1C melanoma. The prognosis tends to worsen from M1A to M1B to M1C.

Table 5-3. The M staging for melanoma

M0 No metastases present	
M1 Metastases present	A: skin and soft tissues only
	B: lungs only
	C: all other organs or elevated LDH

Other Factors

Although they are not taken into consideration for staging purposes, a number of other features may influence the course of melanoma. For instance, part of the white blood cells, called lymphocytes, are thought to be responsible for fighting infections and cancer. Patients seem to have a better outcome and response to treatment when many lymphocytes are in their melanoma lesions. Therefore, if lymphocytes are found in large numbers the prognosis may be better.

Another type of immune system cell, dendritic cells, are the major source of initiating an immune response. Large numbers of such cells have been reported to be a favorable sign. Melanomas with increased numbers of dendritic cells, as when lymphocytes are present, may also make the melanoma cells more susceptible to immune attack. Much research has been focused on learning how to galvanize the immune system to attack melanoma (see Chapters 12 and 13).

Physicians and scientists have been equally intrigued by regression in melanoma specimens. Regression refers to areas of melanoma that appear to be undergoing destruction. At first glance, regression may seem like a good sign and suggests that the immune system may be actively trying to destroy the melanoma. But some researchers have suggested that regression means the melanoma may have been deeper at some time in the past; the melanoma cells may have already gained access to the lymphatic vessels and started to spread before the immune system could control the primary melanoma. The evidence right now seems to favor the latter and so regression is most often considered a bad sign. When I find regression I will often evaluate the lymph nodes for evidence of spread even if the melanoma is less than one millimeter thick.

The location of the melanoma on the body may also influence the prognosis. Melanomas on the arms and legs often have a much better prognosis than melanomas of the head, neck, chest, abdomen, or back. Melanomas of the fingernail beds and those located in the eye or mucous membranes often are more threatening than those on the skin. When it comes to melanoma, men may do worse than women but this has not been substantiated completely. In general, younger patients fare worse than older patients. These factors are not considered for staging purposes but may be important variables in individual cases. For example, I saw a seventeen-year-old boy with a melanoma on his arm that measured 0.8 millimeters deep. Ordinarily I would have simply excised the melanoma. Because of his age and gender, I was more aggressive and evaluated his lymph nodes which fortunately did not have any melanoma.

Clinical Staging

You are probably already familiar with the four clinical stages of cancer, which are noted by roman numerals—I, II, III, and IV for all cancers. The clinical staging system makes things a bit easier to understand and follow; it includes only four stages based on the TNM factors listed in Tables 5-1, 5-2, and 5-3. You may hear your doctor mention these clinical staging terms but always ask about your TNM staging as well because it provides more detail about the extent of your melanoma at the time of diagnosis.

Stages I and II are defined as primary melanomas that have not spread to lymph nodes or other organs. Stage I includes those melanomas that are less than one millimeter thick and those that are one–two millimeters thick without ulceration. Stage II includes melanomas one to two millimeters thick that are ulcerated and any melanoma greater than two millimeters. Since the risk of a melanoma returning and the chances of survival are directly related to the thickness of the melanoma, the distinction between Stage I and II melanoma is significant. Survival is over 90 percent for Stage I melanoma and closer to 80 percent for Stage II melanoma.

Stage III is defined as melanoma involving the local lymph nodes. No matter how thin a melanoma is, if the lymph nodes contain melanoma, a Stage III is automatically applied to the patient. Stage IV means that the melanoma has metastasized to other organs in the body or the LDH is elevated in the blood.

The Melanoma Staging Work-Up

Now that you understand *what* staging consists of, you probably are wondering *how* to find out your own melanoma stage. How the stage of melanoma is determined varies for each of the three variables—the tumor (T), lymph nodes (N), and metastases (M). The treatment of the primary melanoma lesion depends on the T stage. Why? Simply because very thin melanomas are less likely to spread than thick ones. Melanoma confined to the epidermis—T0 or "in situ" melanoma—has no probability of spreading at all and so further work-up is unnecessary. Melanoma lesions less than one millimeter into the dermis are classified as thin melanomas. Simple surgical removal can cure these melanomas. Similarly, a melanoma that is less than one millimeter, or a T1, has a less than 22 percent chance of spreading; so low that further intervention usually is not warranted. I do a further work-up even in very thin melanomas, however, if it's a high-risk patient (for example, a young person or a male) or I notice other high-risk features such as ulceration or tumor regression.

Any melanoma that is greater than 1 millimeter—T2, T3, or T4—or is high risk for other reasons, including most mucosal melanomas, requires the N staging. Lesions that are four millimeters or greater (i.e., T4) also require M staging. First, a physician skilled in examining lymph nodes carefully feels for any enlargements. A needle or surgical biopsy is performed if the doctor encounters any enlarged nodes. If all the lymph nodes feel normal during the physical exam, a surgical procedure called sentinel lymph node mapping is used to detect melanoma in lymph nodes. This procedure (see Chapter 7 for more detail) has largely replaced formal lymph node dissections and can often detect even very small melanoma cells in single lymph nodes.

If the lymph nodes are normal, a metastatic work-up is usually not necessary. In low risk situations a more informal metastatic evaluation may suffice. For this, I typically perform a chest X-ray and measure the liver enzymes, including the LDH, once a year. If the lymph nodes do contain melanoma or if the primary melanoma is deeper than four millimeters, regardless of the lymph node status, a comprehensive metastatic work-up is needed.

A more extensive metastatic work-up is indicated for patients with symptoms of metastatic disease or those with very large melanomas or extensive lymph node involvement. The work-up includes imaging all sites where melanoma may have spread within the body: the brain, chest, abdomen, and pelvis, and the bones. Imaging is usually done through special scans performed by the radiologist, described below. These tests have become quite sensitive and can find melanoma when it is as small as one centimeter and may be easier to treat. In addition to the imaging it is also important to obtain blood tests to determine the liver enzymes, especially the LDH.

MRI Scans

Whenever the possibility of metastatic melanoma exists, the brain is the first place we look. A magnetic resonance imaging scan or MRI is the best method. The MRI employs a combination of a strong magnetic field and radiofrequency waves to provide clear and detailed pictures of the internal organs. MRI has been especially helpful in providing high quality images of the brain and can often distinguish benign from malignant tumors. The MRI requires specialized equipment and physicians trained in conducting and interpreting MRI scans. The MRI scan is usually performed in special radiology departments or clinics. Patients with metal on or in their bodies, such as a pacemaker or a metal plate, cannot have an MRI since the large magnet used will attract all metallic objects when it is turned on. (In situations in which an MRI is not possible, a CT scan with contrast material is the next best thing.) The radiologist examines the MRI and writes a report describing any abnormalities seen on the scan, including lesions, swelling, or bleeding. Melanoma often appears as a "lesion" and the radiologist describes exactly where the lesion is in the brain and how big the lesion measures in two dimensions.

CT Scans

The best way to image the chest, abdomen, and pelvis is with a computed tomography scan or CT scan (also called a CAT scan). In a CT scan, X-rays take a cross-sectional image—or "slice"—through the body while a patient lies still on a table and a machine rotates around 360°. Movement can interfere with the collection of the picture and lead to a distorted image, so if you have a CT scan you must hold very still. The images obtained can be enhanced by the presence of contrast material, such as iodine injected into the veins to allow the blood vessels to be better defined. Similarly, a contrast dye that you swallow prior to the scan appears white on the CT scan images and accumulates in the bowels. The radiologist can distinguish normal bowel from any abnormal masses, which will appear as a darkened area next to the white contrast material. A computer processes the X-ray images into a composite picture, which is displayed on a screen and can be developed as a picture on film. The CT scan is especially useful for finding melanoma because it clearly demonstrates the shape and exact location of any abnormal masses or cancers. The technique can image soft tissues, internal organs, and bones very well (although the MRI is better for the brain). The CT scan is very sensitive for finding melanoma as long as the melanoma is at least 1 centimeter in size or larger. The major drawbacks of CT scans are being uncomfortable lying on a hard table while the pictures are taken and occasional bad reactions or allergic responses to the contrast material used.

Bone Scan

I do not typically use this scan since the CT scan images the bones very well. If you have pain over the bones or there is concern that the CT scan may have missed a particular bone, then a bone scan may be done. Usually performed in the nuclear medicine department of a hospital, a bone scan can evaluate all bones in the body. The scan is done by first injecting a radioactive substance called a radionuclide into the veins. This radionuclide collects in areas where the bone may be destroyed by melanoma cells. The normal bone cells will be overactive to replace the destroyed bone and these overactive cells pick up the radionuclide. The radioactivity can be detected by a gamma camera, an imaging device that detects radiation. The camera can be placed over all areas of the body and detects areas of high bone activity, referred to as "hot spots." Hot spots simply mean that there is activity in the bone at that site, but the presence of melanoma can only be confirmed by a biopsy or clinical judgment. The radioactive substance is rapidly cleared from the body through the urine in about twenty-four hours with no ill effects.

PET Scan

The recently developed PET scan is often used for finding metastatic melanoma. PET (positron emission tomography) locates areas of abnormal function, such as rapidly dividing melanoma cells. Fluoridated sugar molecules are injected into the veins and travel to cells that are actively dividing, as is occurring in sites of melanoma growth. Once inside the melanoma cells, the fluoridated molecule can be detected by a specialized gamma camera just as in a bone scan. The detection is based on having many cells with the tracer in one area and the ability to detect the radionuclide is decreased when the number of cells are few. It is important to lie as still as possible for a PET scan so the sugar molecules do not enter the muscle cells, which could make it difficult to interpret the scan. The PET scan has been close to 95 percent sensitive for finding melanoma cells but is not effective when the melanoma is less than one centimeter in size, so it must be interpreted carefully. The PET scan may also identify other diseases, such as infections; only a biopsy or careful clinical judgment should be used to confirm the PET scan results. An advantage of the PET scan is that it allows an image of the entire body, whereas the CT scan focuses on particular sites. The CT scan provides better anatomical information and measurements of the size of melanoma lesions, however. Therefore, I generally prefer CT scans, as they provide more significant information and concentrate on those areas of the body where melanoma is more likely to be hidden from detection by physical examination.

Table 5-4. Scans and tests for metastatic melanoma

Test	Comments
Magnetic Resonance Imaging (MRI)	Useful for evaluation of the brain and liver
Computed Tomography (CT)	Used for chest, abdomen, and pelvis
Bone scan	Used when specific bone involvement is suspected and not easily seen on CT scan
PET scan	Can detect melanoma in most parts of the body; used as a supplement to CT scans
Ultrasound	Some evidence of benefit for melanoma but not used routinely
Liver enzyme tests	Blood test that measures the level of key liver enzymes in the blood; elevation indicates liver involvement
LDH	Blood test that indicates an especially poor prognosis when elevated
Blood counts and chemistry	Useful for assessing general status of patients and their ability to tolerate treatment

What to Expect If You Are Having a Scan

You should know certain things before going for your test if your doctor orders a scan. Your doctor should explain her rationale for choosing a particular test or tests and explain what she's looking for. Sometimes it is just part of routine staging and nothing is expected to show up. In other cases, the doctor may be searching for a particular problem.

Keep in mind the following tips when undergoing a scan:

- If you are nervous or anxious, ask the radiologist to let you look at the machine ahead of time. Alternatively, you can have a mild sedative before the scan.

- During the scan you lie on a flat table that may move through a "doughnut" type machine. If you are claustrophobic, ask for an open scan, which does not enclose the head. In the case of a bone or PET scan, the machine may revolve around your table.

- Tell your doctor if you have an allergy to iodine, contrast dye, or shellfish as this may make it more likely that you will react to the contrast dyes used in CT scans.

- In some cases intravenous contrast or radionuclides require that an IV catheter be placed in the arm just prior to the scan. This is usually no more painful than a simple needle stick for blood drawing, but if you're sensitive to being jabbed, you should ask ahead of time.

- Avoid wearing clothing that contains metal, such as zippers, and remove all metallic objects before the scan, including rings, bracelets, necklaces, hairpins, coins, and keys. Before the test, you change into a gown, which prevents metal in clothing from interfering with the scan.

- Ask how long you should avoid food or drink on the day of your scan if you require oral contrast. Tell the radiologist if you are a diabetic so they can advise you on when to take your regular medications.

- Go to the bathroom before the test to prevent interrupting the scan before it is completed.

- For nearly all scans you will be asked to keep as still as possible since any movement—even breathing—can result in blurry images. You need to hold your breath for a few seconds when the scanner is taking pictures.

- Once the scan is completed, drink plenty of water to flush the contrast material from your body.

- Shortness of breath, a rapid heartbeat, diarrhea, stomach upset, a new rash, or hives are all delayed reactions to the dye. Notify your doctor immediately if you experience any of these effects.

- It is helpful to have someone with you during the test for moral support and to drive you home when the test is done.

Scans using dyes take more time to complete, but most scans are usually done in about one to two hours. You'll spend between twenty minutes to an hour actually in the scanner, depending on how fast the machine is. Chances are slim that you will receive the scan results on the spot. The scan is developed and then sent to a radiologist for expert review and opinion. The radiologist generates and sends a written report to the referring physician. This process can take up to one week to complete. In the event of a serious finding the referring physician is usually notified immediately, however, so no news may be good news. I like to have my patients come back to the office once the results are in so we can go through them carefully and discuss what each one means.

*   *   *

Now THAT YOU KNOW the stages of melanoma and the procedures used to determine the stage, you may be feeling overwhelmed by so much information. The good news is that most patients I see have Stage I or II melanomas that can usually be cured with surgical removal. Some patients have Stage III melanoma and only a few have developed Stage IV melanoma at diagnosis. You'll appreciate the importance of staging when I discuss the treatment options for melanoma in the next chapters. You will see that it is critical to know about the stage and implement effective treatment as soon as possible. If you understand the stage of melanoma, a logical plan for therapy can be developed.

Columbia Melanoma Center Case Studies

Wendy, a seventy-nine-year-old woman, went to her dermatologist about a small mole on her left upper back that had increased in size over the preceding six months. The dermatologist performed a biopsy in the office and found a melanoma 4.5 millimeters deep but without ulceration. Wendy, who was otherwise healthy, came to the Melanoma Center for evaluation. Although I did not feel any lymph nodes under her left arm or in her neck, I ordered a metastatic work-up before proceeding with any further treatment because the melanoma was so deep.

The metastatic work-up included blood counts, chemistry, and liver enzymes, which were all normal. An MRI of the brain also was normal. A CT scan of the chest, however, revealed the presence of many lung tumors, which were melanoma metastases consistent with spread of the melanoma to the lungs. A melanoma in the right adrenal gland showed up on the abdominal CT scan. Based on these findings, I started Wendy on systemic immunotherapy. She is tolerating treatment well.

Wendy's case is an excellent example of why staging melanoma is so important. Her treatment changed dramatically once we knew the

melanoma had spread. A less experienced physician might have simply removed her skin melanoma and never realized she had melanoma in the
lungs and adrenal gland. Through the staging procedures I was able to
quickly detect the spread of melanoma and start appropriate treatment.

Ask Your Doctor

If you are diagnosed with melanoma that may need to be staged, ask
the following questions:

1. *What is the depth of my melanoma?* This is the most important
   information for staging and treatment purposes for the primary
   melanoma. Melanoma is considered thin (less than one millimeter),
   intermediate (one–four millimeters), or thick (greater than four
   millimeters). Thin melanomas are more easily cured with surgical
   removal. Intermediate melanomas require assessment of the local or
   nearby lymph nodes, and thick melanomas require a metastatic work-
   up before treatment.
2. *Is there any ulceration in my melanoma?* Ulceration, or absence of
   overlying skin, is the second most important feature of the primary
   melanoma. Ulceration means the melanoma is more serious and
   requires attention by a melanoma specialist.
3. *Based on the biopsy report, what is my prognosis?* The biopsy
   reports the thickness of the melanoma and the presence of
   ulceration. In general, the thinner the melanoma the better the
   prognosis. Although this information may be helpful, it does not
   necessarily take into account the status of the lymph nodes or
   internal organs, and knowledge of whether or not melanoma has
   spread to these sites may be necessary to fully determine the
   prognosis for patients who have intermediate or thick melanoma
   lesions. Based on the biopsy report further staging may be
   necessary to evaluate the lymph nodes and internal organs. Even
   given a bad prognosis, patients often respond well to therapy.
4. *Did you find any enlarged lymph nodes when you examined me?* The
   local lymph nodes must be evaluated in melanoma patients,

especially if the melanoma is greater than one millimeter deep. The easiest way to do this is to have your doctor examine the related lymph node areas for enlarged nodes. A needle biopsy or surgical biopsy should be performed to confirm melanoma.

5. *Did you find anything else abnormal?* A health care professional can often detect signs of melanoma spread during a physical exam, which should be performed before other more expensive tests. The examination may lead to further testing; for example, if the doctor finds tenderness over the bones when he examines you, he may order a bone scan.

6. *Do I need additional treatment?* Your doctor will only be able to answer this question once the staging is completed.

7. *Do I need a chest X-ray?* An annual chest X-ray is generally recommended for all patients at intermediate risk for recurrent melanoma. In my practice every patient with an intermediate or thick melanoma has annual chest X-rays unless CT scans are performed.

8. *Do I need to have a CT scan of my chest, abdomen, and pelvis?* All patients with melanomas greater than four millimeters thick and/or melanoma in the lymph nodes should have these CT scans. A baseline scan should be done once to document that there is no spread of melanoma. These scans may be repeated every three months if melanoma is detected or less frequently depending on the results of the staging work-up. Ask your doctor about how often you should repeat these scans.

9. *Do I need an MRI scan of my brain?* Same criteria as for CT scans: All patients with melanomas greater than four millimeters thick and/or melanoma in the lymph nodes should get an MRI of the brain.

10. *Do I need to have a PET scan?* You may need a PET scan in situations where the CT scans and MRI are equivocal or difficult to interpret, or if the CT scan or MRI cannot easily visualize suspected melanoma in a certain area. I often use the PET scan for patients with one site of metastatic disease before recommending surgery to remove the melanoma.

11. *Do I need blood work done?* Routine blood counts and chemistry

values should be obtained at least annually for most patients with melanoma. The liver enzyme tests are especially important for demonstrating melanoma in the liver.

12. *Do I need to have my LDH level tested?* The LDH test, a blood test that is highly predictive of melanoma metastasis, is an integral part of melanoma staging today. All melanoma patients should be tested annually or more frequently depending on the stage of disease.

13. *Are there any abnormal findings in my blood tests or X-rays?* It is your right to know the results of any of these tests. Ask your doctor to review the pertinent findings and explain their importance. You need to understand the results and have any uncertainties explained or cleared up before choosing your therapy.

14. *Do I need any further tests?* If there are any uncertainties then additional testing may be necessary. Occasionally scans or blood tests may uncover problems not related to melanoma. If you need to have more tests these should be scheduled quickly; ask when they will be done. It is important to move on and avoid long delays before starting definitive treatment for your melanoma.

15. *Do I need to see a specialist in melanoma surgery or oncology?* If you have a more advanced stage of melanoma, you will be referred to a specialist. In general, a surgical oncologist cares for Stage III melanoma patients, while the medical oncologist usually is called on for Stage III and IV patients.

16. *When do I need to come back?* After you have been told your test results and the stage of your melanoma you will need to return for definitive treatment. Ask your doctor when treatment will start and who will be coordinating your care.

PART THREE

Treating Melanoma

CHAPTER SIX

How Do You Treat Primary Melanoma (Stages I and II)?

THE TREATMENT OF primary melanoma (Stage I and II) is surgical excision or removal of all melanoma cells in order to halt its spread. Without treatment, the natural course for melanoma is to grow into deeper layers from its most common primary site, the skin. Once it reaches the mid- to lower dermis, melanoma cells can enter the lymphatic vessels and spread to the local lymph nodes. From the lymph nodes melanoma can then spread to virtually any other organ in the body. In cases where complete removal is possible and no spread has occurred, melanoma can be cured.

Wide Local Excision

The surgical treatment is a wide local excision, in which the entire melanoma and surrounding skin are removed. Exactly how wide is "wide"? The answer depends on how deep into the skin the melanoma has grown. This is an important point; it is not how large the melanoma grows across the surface of the skin but how deep it goes into the dermis that determines the extent of surgery. Therefore, a melanoma relatively large in circumference on the surface of the skin may require less treatment than a tiny nodule that has grown deep into the underlying dermis below the surface of the skin.

The margin, or amount of surrounding skin to be removed as part of a wide local excision, has been the subject of much debate for many years. A large number of clinical studies have compared different margins of skin removal to determine the chances of melanoma returning as well as the chances of living a normal life after the operation. The good news is that over time we have learned that for most melanoma lesions a smaller margin may lead to an equally positive prognosis as a wider margin. The general guidelines that I use are as follows (see Figure 6-1):

- Early melanomas that have not gone deeper than the epidermis, also called in-situ melanoma: a margin of 0.5 centimeters, or about a quarter of an inch.

- Melanomas less than one millimeter deep: a margin of one centimeter, or about half an inch.

- Any melanoma deeper than one millimeter: a margin of two centimeters, or about one inch.

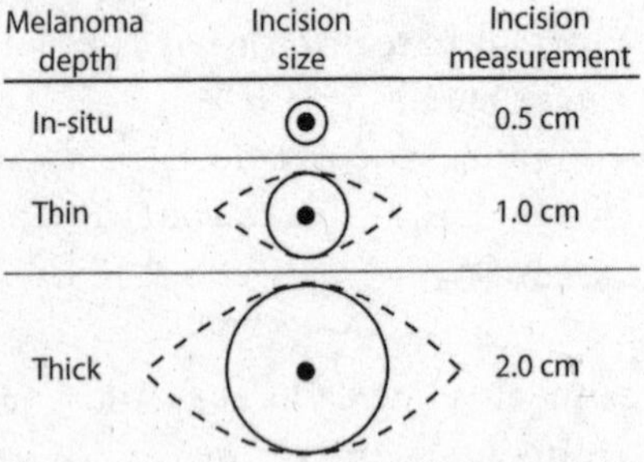

Melanoma depth	Incision size	Incision measurement
In-situ	⊙	0.5 cm
Thin	< (•) >	1.0 cm
Thick	< (•) >	2.0 cm

Figure 6-1. Margins for melanomas of different depths

Although Figure 6-1 shows the margins as a circle, the actual incision shape most surgeons use is an ellipse (see dotted line). This shape allows the skin to close back more easily, without the skin having to stretch much. The closure of any surgical incision without tension results in better healing and less scar formation. Although I can usually close the skin with no problem, sometimes there is some tension or the margins are large enough to cause a major defect. For example, when the primary melanoma is very large in circumference—if a melanoma is four centimeters across and a two centimeter margin is necessary on all sides—the total skin removal will be eight centimeters. While it may still be easy to close if the melanoma is on the back or abdominal wall, it can be difficult if it is on the face or knee cap. In the event that the defect is large we have some tricks that can be used to help bring the skin together, including larger and stronger stitches, a special technique called undermining, or even a skin graft.

An important point: When a melanoma is quite small the entire melanoma may be removed with the biopsy procedure, but *this is not adequate treatment*. If you are suspected of having melanoma, a biopsy is performed to confirm the diagnosis and determine the depth of the melanoma. This information is then used to plan the real treatment procedure—the wide local excision. If you have only had a biopsy, I do not consider the melanoma to have been treated adequately. The biopsy is necessary to determine how deep the melanoma has grown, since this information is used to plan the size of the margins needed as part of the wide local excision.

While many dermatologists are comfortable performing small excisions for melanoma, if the lesion is deep you may need to see a surgical oncologist for treatment. A plastic surgeon might also be needed when complicated closures are required following an excision. It is important to ascertain whether your doctor is familiar with these procedures and whether they perform them frequently. A biopsy is relatively straightforward and simple. Definitive treatment requires a higher level of expertise.

The operation may require that you have some routine blood tests to make sure there are no problems with bleeding or any of the major organ systems. A chest X-ray and EKG before surgery are also fairly standard, especially if you have any other medical problems.

The surgical procedure is performed either in an office area dedicated to surgery or in a hospital operating room. Many times the excision can be done under local anesthetic, although for larger lesions a stronger anesthetic may be recommended. After the skin is numbed with the anesthetic or the patient is put to sleep, an incision is made with a scalpel. When I perform this operation I first draw the margins on all sides with a ruler and a marking pen right on the skin. The incision is usually an ellipse that encompasses the widest margins and extends a little bit on either side of the margins to enable closure. Once the skin is divided, it is critical to remove all layers of the skin and the immediate layer of fat just under the skin. After the specimen is removed, I make sure there is no bleeding or any other unusual masses in the wound.

The next step is to bring the skin back together and close the incision. If the skin comes together easily I use a suture that leaves little scar; the stitches dissolve on their own in about six to eight weeks.

If the skin does not come together easily, the edges may require some loosening up through a technique called undermining, whereby the tissue just below the skin on all sides is divided to free the movement of the overlying skin. This often does the trick and the skin can be closed with stronger, non-dissolving stitches. These require removal after seven to ten days.

If the skin still does not close, then a skin graft or flap closure is needed. This can usually be anticipated before the operation so both patient and doctor are prepared. A skin graft involves removing a very thin layer of skin from another site on the body, usually the lateral thigh. This healthy skin can be stretched and then placed over the site of the removed skin. Skin grafts take a little longer to heal but eventually fully cover the area. In some cases a flap of muscle and skin can be used to cover a large area where a skin graft might not work, such as on the face or near the bend of the knee. A plastic surgeon is often called on to perform complex flap closures.

The major complications of wide local excision are similar to other types of minor surgery: bleeding and infection. I tell my patients that even with the best operation there is always the possibility that the melanoma will come back, although this is very rare with adequate margins. There also are no guarantees against scarring since everyone heals differently. In most cases the scar is very minor and often heals well within several months.

People with medical problems, such as heart disease, diabetes mellitus, and obesity, may be prone to other complications. Your primary doctor should be aware that you are having melanoma surgery and may suggest extra precautions. He may put you on antibiotics before the operation to help prevent infection, or take measures to prevent blood clots in the legs after surgery.

The surgical incision usually heals within seven to ten days. The surgeon will want to see you then, to make sure that the incision has healed well and that there are no signs of infection. Your doctor will then review the results of the pathology report with you. The pathologist will confirm that the entire melanoma was removed, that the margins were free of tumor cells, and will report how deeply the melanoma extended and whether there was ulceration present. If the depth is different from the biopsy additional therapy may be necessary. Ultimately, it is the thickness of melanoma that determines the extent of treatment.

Other Treatment Options for Primary Melanoma

Although wide local excision is the treatment of choice for melanoma, there are other treatment options that may be used in selected cases. Discuss them carefully with your doctor since most of these procedures result in the direct destruction of the melanoma within the skin and do not allow a careful pathology review.

Radiation Therapy

Radiation is not commonly used because it does not allow direct examination of the lesion, clear margins cannot be accurately predicted, and the complications are generally more severe than those seen with surgical excision. Nevertheless, there are times when radiation may be very useful as a primary or secondary treatment. Contrary to popular opinion, melanoma cells may be quite sensitive to radiation. Radiation therapy can be used to kill melanoma on the skin and in other sites. I sometimes use radiation for patients with very large melanomas where an operation would result in disfiguring defects. Radiation may also be useful for patients who have a large number of melanoma lesions, which prevents simple excision of the skin. It may take up to two years for melanoma lesions to disappear after radiation treatment. The decision to use radiation should be made on an individual basis and requires discussion between the oncologist, surgeon, and radiation oncologist, who actually performs the procedure.

Laser Therapy

Laser is an acronym that stands for "Light Amplification by Stimulated Emission of Radiation." First developed in the 1960s, laser technology uses either a solid or gas medium that when stimulated induces electromagnetic radiation in the visible light or infrared spectrum. Lasers are used in the medical field to provide a highly focused beam that results in a photothermal effect and vaporizes tissue on contact. The use of laser therapy has little pain and swelling compared to other techniques. Laser therapy has been proposed for the treatment of skin cancers other than melanoma and may be quite useful for small benign tumors. There is little evidence that laser therapy is appropriate for melanoma, however. The major problem with laser therapy is that no tissue is obtained for evaluation and there is no way to confirm that all the melanoma cells have been destroyed. I do not recommend laser therapy for the treatment of primary melanoma except in highly specific circumstances, such as for very small melanomas in patients who cannot have surgery.

Cryotherapy

Cryotherapy uses extreme cold to freeze tumor cells and has been useful for some types of cancer. This technique suffers from the same problems as laser therapy and has not been validated for the treatment of melanoma.

Mohs Micrographic Surgery

Mohs technique was popularized for the treatment of basal cell carcinomas, a more benign skin cancer. Mohs involves the sequential removal of a tumor with immediate microscopic examination to determine if tumor cells are present. The dissection continues as long as the tumor is still present in the specimen. The technique is especially useful for basal cell carcinomas because it allows the complete removal of the tumor without taking any additional skin. This leads to an optimal cosmetic result since the minimum amount of tissue is removed. Mohs technique is not recommended for melanoma since a wide margin is necessary. The other issue is that melanoma cells are more difficult to detect on frozen tissue examination as used in the Mohs technique. Mohs technique needs to be tested further before it can be recommended for melanoma treatment.

Topical Chemotherapy

To date there has been no effective topical chemotherapy for the treatment of melanoma.

Aldara Cream

Aldara cream is a synthetic substance used for treating common skin warts and basal cell carcinoma. The substance in Aldara cream activates dendritic skin cells to produce interferons and other cytokines that may activate a strong local immune response against the melanoma cells. The reaction looks and feels like an inflammation on the skin, which reddens.

The melanoma either turns into a scab and sloughs off, or is absorbed by the body. Although it is still experimental, there is some evidence that Aldara cream may be useful for the treatment of small, thin melanomas. More research needs to be done to see exactly how effective Aldara cream is; the approach also prevents pathologic review of the specimen. If Aldara is beneficial in further clinical testing it may play a role in selected cases of small melanoma lesions.

Now YOU UNDERSTAND why it is so important to find melanoma when it is still small. Early diagnosis can mean complete eradication of the melanoma by simple surgical excision. Constant vigilance, including monthly self-examination and regular dermatology screening, can lead to successful treatment for most melanomas.

Columbia Melanoma Center Case Studies

Sam, a fifty-five-year-old, had a pigmented mole on the top of his scalp for many years. His wife noticed that the mole had begun to grow and turn darker over the last three months. The mole measured six centimeters and was shaped in an irregular circle. Melanoma was diagnosed after his dermatologist did a biopsy. He found a superficial spreading melanoma 1.85 millimeters deep without any areas of ulceration.

When Sam came to the Melanoma Center for treatment, I explained that he needed a wide local excision with a two-centimeter skin margin. I excised the lesion and removed two centimeters of additional skin. This left a large gap approximately ten centimeters across on an area of skin that is difficult to stretch. I placed a skin graft from his thigh over the defect on his scalp. One week later the graft was healing nicely and I took out his sutures. The pathology report indicated that all the melanoma had been removed and that there were no areas deeper than the 1.85 millimeters seen on the original biopsy report.

After four weeks the graft had healed and Sam was feeling very well. We set up clinic visits every three months for the next year to examine his skin. I instructed him to avoid prolonged sun exposure or use protective clothing and sunscreen when outside.

Sam is typical of a patient whose large area of excision is in a part of the body that is difficult to close. The skin graft in this case was simple and healed quickly. Although hair will not grow on a skin graft site, Sam was already partially balding and did not mind. He wears a hat to cover his scalp most of the time and continues to be free of melanoma.

Ask Your Doctor

If you need to be treated for Stage I or II melanoma, ask the following questions:

1. *How wide will the wide local excision be?* The margins of a wide local excision depend on how deep the primary melanoma is on the biopsy report. The deeper the melanoma, the wider the margin of resection must be to prevent recurrence and spread of disease.

2. *What are the complications of wide local excision?* There may be complications, other than bleeding or infection, depending on where on the body the melanoma is located and how deep it has grown. Always ask your surgeon about potential complications of both the operation and the anesthesia prior to signing a consent form.

3. *How often will I be seen following the procedure?* It is customary to be seen at least once after the operation to make certain that the surgical site is healing well and to review the pathology report. You may need to be seen more frequently and should ask when to return for routine evaluation and follow-up.

4. *How many melanoma resections have you done?* Most surgeons do not mind when patients seek information. The wide local excision, the procedure performed for melanoma, is very important and may influence your outcome later. Be as confident as possible that your surgeon is competent at melanoma surgery and understands the management of this disease.

5. *What is the local recurrence rate for melanoma at this site?* When adequate margins are obtained at the time of the operation for melanoma, the risk of recurrence is usually extremely low. If the margins are compromised because of an anatomical consideration, or the melanoma is very deep, the chance of recurrence may be higher. Ask your surgeon if more frequent follow-up is needed in the situation where recurrence may be higher.

6. *What is the risk that the melanoma has spread to other sites?* Like all other decisions in melanoma treatment this depends on the depth of the primary melanoma. Other features include the location of the lesion on the body, the sex of the patient, the presence of ulceration in the melanoma, and the age of the patient. If the risk of spread is high, additional studies and treatments may be necessary.

7. *Will I need additional treatment?* This will likely depend on the results of the initial pathology report describing how deep the melanoma has grown and whether there is ulceration in the lesion. Since evaluation of the local lymph nodes can usually be done at the same time as wide local excision, it is helpful to see if this is necessary. Likewise, if there is a high probability for distant spread, additional imaging scans may be indicated prior to surgery.

CHAPTER SEVEN

How Do You Treat Melanoma in the Lymph Nodes?

MOST STAGE I AND II MELANOMAS will be cured through surgical removal. In cases where the melanoma has already spread, simple surgical removal is not enough to completely eradicate the melanoma from the body. Melanoma that has spread but is confined to the lymph nodes is called Stage III melanoma. In this chapter, I will explain how we determine and treat Stage III melanoma.

Why Are Lymph Nodes Significant in Melanoma?

The body has thousands of lymph nodes, which are normally small marble-size balls, approximately one centimeter in diameter. These pieces of tissue contain a collection of cells involved in the immune system. The lymph nodes serve to warn the body that an infection is present. If a bacterial infection occurs, lymph nodes start a complex process referred to as an immune response. The immune response organizes an attack on any invading organism, such as a bacteria or virus. The lymph nodes may swell up when they are starting an immune response, and you may notice the swollen lymph nodes if you have an infection: for example, "swollen glands" in the neck after a bad sore throat or upper respiratory tract infection. When the infection ends, the "glands"—lymph nodes—disappear. Lymph nodes can be called on over and over again to help fight infections.

While lymph nodes can be located throughout the body, some areas have a large number of lymph nodes and are referred to as lymph node basins. The most prominent lymph node basins are in the neck, under both arms, and in the groin. Lymph nodes in the neck protect against infections that enter the body through the face, mouth, nose, and ears. The lymph nodes under the arm protect against infections that may enter through the skin or blood vessels of the arms. The lymph nodes of the groin protect against similar infections that may enter the body through the legs or feet. You won't be surprised to learn that lymph nodes in the chest and abdomen likely protect against infections trying to enter the body through the lungs or intestines.

Why mention infection-fighting lymph nodes in a book about melanoma? Most cancers, including melanoma, actually spread from their original site through specialized vessels, similar to blood vessels, that bring the cancer cells directly to the lymph nodes. In fact, for nearly every kind of cancer (there are some exceptions), the lymph nodes are the first place where cancer spreads. Scientists do not entirely understand why this is the case, but some investigators believe that the lymph nodes may fight cancer cells, much as they fight invading bacterial or viral infections. Whatever the reason, we do know that the number of involved lymph nodes is an important factor in survival, and we now know that the single most important determining feature for patients with melanoma is whether melanoma is even in a single lymph node. Although there is some variation, most physicians believe that nearly half of all melanoma patients with lymph node involvement will not survive longer than five years. Therefore, finding out if the lymph nodes contain melanoma and applying appropriate treatment as soon as possible is key to a patient's recovery.

Identifying Melanoma in Lymph Nodes

The only way to be certain that melanoma has or has not spread to a lymph node is for a trained pathologist to examine the lymph node under a microscope. The problem is that given the number of lymph nodes in the body, it is difficult or even impossible to examine all of them! Fortunately, new technical procedures can identify single lymph nodes that are more likely to have melanoma if indeed the melanoma cells have spread.

There is no chance that melanomas contained only in the epidermis have spread, and so the chances of finding melanoma in a lymph node is practically zero. My only caveat is that sometimes melanomas may regress, or shrink, in the skin. If the biopsy or surgical removal is done after the regression, it is possible that the melanoma had spread during the time it was deeper in the skin. When a pathologist reports signs of such regressing melanomas, I usually try to check the lymph nodes to be certain that no spread has occurred.

Thin melanomas that are less than one millimeter deep in the skin have less than a 2 percent chance of spreading. Clinical studies show that certain characteristics of the melanoma may indicate those at an increased risk of lymph node involvement. Melanomas with areas of regression or ulceration, or located on the head, neck, or trunk are more likely to have spread. I will look for lymph node spread in any patient with a melanoma that is greater than 0.75 millimeters with any of these features. Otherwise, I only look for lymph node spread in patients with a melanoma deeper than one millimeter.

If a lymph node is swollen and can be felt by the patient or doctor, there is usually little doubt about the presence of melanoma in the lymph node: 90 percent of patients with a known skin melanoma and a swollen lymph node have Stage III melanoma. Either a needle biopsy or a surgical biopsy of the lymph node can confirm it. Treatment is a surgical procedure called a lymph node dissection, which I will describe in more detail below.

Sentinel Nodes

Is there a way to find the affected lymph nodes earlier, before they enlarge? When I was a medical student, the only known way to do this was to remove and examine all the lymph nodes near the melanoma. Today we have a better method: the sentinel lymph node biopsy. This procedure is rapidly becoming the standard operation for patients with intermediate or thick melanomas, or anyone with a risk of melanoma spreading to the lymph nodes.

The sentinel node biopsy incorporates our knowledge of how melanoma spreads to nearby lymph nodes with new techniques to identify the individual, diseased lymph nodes. Although the procedure is revolutionizing how we treat patients with melanoma, we need to wait for the results of several large clinical studies now in progress to fully determine the benefit of the procedure.

Sentinel node biopsy is based on the fact that melanoma cells enter the local lymphatic vessels in the skin and then travel through these vessels until they encounter a lymph node. The lymphatic vessel infiltrates the lymph node, and the melanoma gets stuck and begins to grow in the lymph node. The sentinel node is the first lymph node that the melanoma cells reach. What happens next is controversial, but many investigators believe that, once in, the sentinel node melanoma (if not removed) will spread to other lymph nodes and then to internal organs. Therefore, if we can find the sentinel node before it becomes enlarged or swollen, we may be able to prevent any further spread of the melanoma by removing it. Sometimes it is obvious where the lymph node is located—for example melanomas on the thigh will almost always be found in the groin. However, for melanomas on the head, neck, upper abdomen, or back, it can be difficult to predict which lymph nodes may be involved. Using sentinel node procedure results in the proper identification of the sentinel node. In the early stages before the node enlarges, the lymph node is too small to feel by touch. We need another way to find it.

The sentinel node biopsy involves two steps. First, we identify the lymphatic drainage from the original melanoma and the sentinel node by injecting a microscopic protein that is coupled with a small radioactive tracer at the site of the original melanoma. The most commonly used proteins are sulfur colloid and albumin. Once the tracer is injected into the skin, the proteins enter the lymphatic vessels near the melanoma and take the same pathway the melanoma cells take to the first lymph node. The radioactive tracer provides a way to find the hidden lymph node. A gamma camera placed over the outside of the body will light up where the radioactive tracer ends up—the sentinel node. This process is called *lymphoscintigraphy* and is usually performed in the nuclear medicine department before surgery. The physician places an "X" over the site of the sentinel node so that the surgeon can perform a minor operation removing only one lymph node through a small incision. This is clearly better than removing all the lymph nodes, which was commonly done in the past and frequently subjected people to unnecessary surgery with significant side effects. The surgeon can also use a small hand-held gamma probe to help locate the lymph node in the operating room. The amount of radioactive material used is very small and there is little harm since the lymph node will be removed shortly after the injection anyway.

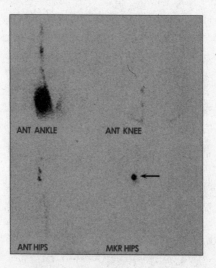

Figure 7-1. Lymphoscintigraphy

Figure 7-1 is an example of a typical lymphoscintigraphic "picture" that is obtained before the operation. The patient was a woman with a deep melanoma on her left foot. She came to the hospital on the morning of her melanoma operation and went to the nuclear medicine department, where they injected a radiotracer protein into the skin around the melanoma on her foot. Two hours after the injection, a gamma camera took this picture, which shows one lymph node in her left groin (arrow). An "X" was placed over this lymph node, so I could find the sentinel node using a very small incision (less than two inches). The sentinel node had no melanoma cells, and I successfully removed the melanoma from her foot. She has been free of melanoma for the past five years and lives a normal life with her daughter and grandchildren.

Another technique to find the sentinel node involves injecting blue dye around the melanoma. Like the radiotracer, it follows the lymphatic vessels to the sentinel node. The dyes then turn the lymph node blue, providing the surgeon with another clue as to where the lymph node is located. A small number of patients may have blue-stained skin for a few months, blue urine for a few days, and in rare cases allergic reactions to the dye. Many surgeons will use both radioactive tracer and the blue dye to be certain that the sentinel node is found, and there is evidence that the accuracy of the procedure is better when both techniques are used.

Sentinel Node Biopsy

If you are having a sentinel node biopsy, you can expect to be in the operating room for under an hour. The procedure, although technically sophisticated, is generally simple in the hands of a surgeon experienced in the operation. It can be done with a local anesthetic, although I often add some stronger anesthetic if there are several nodes or if they are located in a deep position. Next, I make a small incision over the area of the sentinel node. I confirm the location of the sentinel node by finding radioactivity in the lymph node and/or a blue appearance. I remove the lymph node and take a quick look around to make sure that there are no other lymph nodes with radiotracer or blue dye. It is common to find more than one lymph node; these can usually be removed easily at the same time. Recovery is usually rapid. The few side effects include bleeding and infection. Recurrent melanoma at the original melanoma site is also possible, although, based on some reported studies, this risk may be extremely low.

A sentinel node biopsy is best performed when the original melanoma is still in place on the skin, so that the radiotracer and dye can be injected exactly around the melanoma site. It also makes it more likely that the normal lymphatic vessels are intact and will provide access to the lymphatic vessels used by the melanoma cells, if they have spread. Once a melanoma is removed, or shaved, the lymphatic vessels may be disrupted and may decrease the efficacy of the procedure, yet another reason to find a melanoma expert as soon as possible after the diagnosis is made. Typically, only surgical oncologists or general surgeons perform sentinel node biopsies.

The pathologist carefully examines the removed sentinel node. This evaluation is important. Pathologists have several techniques of their own for finding melanoma cells that may be very few in number and hard to detect. In order to better identify the melanoma cells in a piece of lymph node, pathologists stain the cells with a dye. In addition, most pathologists have specialized stains that will cause a color reaction only when specific melanoma proteins are present. The two most commonly used stains, S100 and HMB-45, can sometimes identify cells when they are not readily visible with the standard stains. An even more sensitive technique, called polymerase chain reaction (or PCR), uses molecular probes to find melanoma genes in the lymph nodes. PCR apparently can detect one cell in a million—but whether or not this degree of detection is actually helpful in treating melanoma is being hotly debated.

The pathologist's report will state that there is melanoma present or that there is no melanoma present in the sentinel node. If no melanoma cells are identified, the risk of melanoma spread to the rest of the body is very low, generally considered less than 2 percent, and no further treatment is necessary. This allows us to breathe a sigh of relief and avoid unnecessary operations. If the sentinel node does contain melanoma cells, additional treatment is needed. Melanoma in the sentinel node—or a lymph node—means the patient has Stage III melanoma.

Treatment of Lymph Nodes in Stage III Melanoma

Treatment is a lymph node dissection: a surgical removal of the entire lymph node area. Whether lymph node dissection provides a survival benefit when the lymph nodes are clearly enlarged and can be felt is still controversial, but there is no question that surgery reduces local pain, swelling, and other symptoms. The operation also reveals how many lymph nodes are involved with melanoma, which is valuable prognostic information.

A lymph node dissection is a larger operation than sentinel node biopsy and often requires staying in the hospital for a few days, depending on which lymph node basin is involved. In the case of melanoma on the leg, the lymph nodes are almost always in the groin, although a small number of patients may have lymph nodes behind the knee involved. For groin lymph nodes the procedure is called an *inguinal lymph node dissection* and is usually performed with general anesthesia or spinal anesthesia to make sure there is no sensation from the lower abdomen down through the leg. In a *superficial inguinal lymph node dissection* all the lymph nodes found below the inguinal ligament (the crease between the lower abdomen and the thigh) and above the femoral blood vessels (the large blood vessels to the leg) are removed. I like to use a more vertical incision since it produces better healing and less swelling than horizontal incisions. Typically, there are about ten to fifteen lymph nodes in this area and all are removed. Since the lymphatic vessels are cut during the procedure, a small drain is placed in the incision to allow the lymph fluid to drain for several days. The drain is easily slipped out after a few days and the incision should heal nicely. A *deep inguinal lymph node dissection* includes the removal of the same lymph nodes as in a superficial lymph node dissection as well as deeper lymph nodes located in the pelvis. Obviously this is a longer operation but can usually be done from the same incision. Some surgical oncologists believe that deep node dissection may be beneficial, although there is no proof that this prolongs survival over superficial node dissections. Others think the presence of melanoma in the pelvic lymph nodes indicates more advanced spread and that surgical removal will not provide any benefit. All surgeons do agree that the deep inguinal lymph node dissection has a higher degree of side effects. I believe that the decision to perform a superficial or deep node dissection must be individualized for each patient. If, for example, the surgeon finds melanoma has spread elsewhere, a deep lymph node dissection may not be worthwhile.

For melanomas in the arms or hands the most common lymph node basin is under the arm, or the axillary node basin. A small number of patients may also have lymph nodes involved with melanoma near the elbow. An *axillary lymph node dissection* procedure is similar to the inguinal lymph node dissection and requires general anesthesia. An incision is usually made in the lower portion of the armpit and all lymph nodes found below the axillary vein and between the pectoralis and latissimus muscles are removed. I also remove those lymph nodes found between the pectoralis muscles. There are usually more lymph nodes located in the axilla than in the inguinal basin—approximately fifteen to twenty lymph nodes. A small drain is also placed and the recovery period is similar to that for an inguinal node dissection.

For melanomas involving the head and neck regions the procedure of choice is a *modified radical neck dissection*. This involves removal of the lymph nodes in the front part of the neck extending from the midline near the trachea or windpipe to the area just in front of the ear. Only lymph nodes and very small salivary glands are removed. Since the neck has several important structures that can lead to serious impairments, there have been many studies documenting that leaving these structures intact does not compromise the ability of the operation to remove all cancer cells. In particular, the muscles, large blood vessels, and nerves can be left in place. While it is usually obvious which side of the neck is involved with melanoma, this distinction can be difficult for melanomas that occur near the middle of the face or scalp. Once again, lymphoscintigraphy can be useful although it is often more difficult to identify the sentinel node in this location. Likewise, in some patients, especially those with melanomas located on the back of the scalp, the cancer can spread to the back of the neck and require a slightly different operation to remove these posterior neck lymph nodes. The number of lymph nodes in the neck is higher than anywhere else; it can often be thirty or more. The recovery and use of drains is similar to that of other lymph node dissections.

When a melanoma is located on the chest, abdomen, or back it can often be difficult to predict which nodal basin will be the drainage site for the melanoma. The advent of lymphoscintigraphy has provided a more objective technique for determining the nodal basins at risk and can help to direct the surgeon to the appropriate site. Nonetheless, significant clinical judgment is often needed to make sure that the appropriate nodal basin is dissected in the case of melanomas located near the midline of the body.

Lymph node dissections generally produce similar side effects no matter where the nodal basin is located, although the likelihood of any side effects is highest with inguinal node dissections. The most common side effects are infection, delayed healing of the incision, swelling due to accumulation of lymphatic fluid (*lymphocele*), and bleeding and collection of old blood (*hematoma*). It is not uncommon to have some minor damage to the skin's nerves, leaving patients with small areas of numbness in the arm or thigh. Long-term complications may include swelling of the extremity, which is much more common in the legs, localized pain, and blood clots.

There is remarkably little post-operative pain, and even the pain that occurs dissipates within a few days of the procedure. Patients must limit arm or leg motion for a few weeks, before gradually resuming normal activity.

For those patients whose melanoma is identified by sentinel node biopsy the benefits of a lymph node dissection are not well defined. However, it is possible that the earlier detection of melanoma may lead to a better outcome for patients than when the melanoma is found by enlarged lymph nodes on a physical examination. There are several large clinical studies trying to answer the question of how beneficial lymph node dissection will be after a sentinel node biopsy. At the present time I strongly recommend that all patients with melanoma in their sentinel nodes consider having a lymph node dissection.

Melanoma of Unknown Primary Site

In 2 percent of patients with melanoma, the original, or primary, melanoma site is unknown. These individuals are diagnosed when a doctor identifies melanoma within a lymph node. Most experts believe that the primary melanoma, in such cases, has regressed completely, likely due to an effective immune response. Treatment is nevertheless necessary because the melanoma has spread to lymph nodes before regression is complete. Patients in this special situation inexplicably seem to do the same or even better than those patients whose primary skin melanoma can be found. Treatment is the same and lymph node dissection is recommended as long as no evidence suggests melanoma has spread to other organs.

In-transit Melanoma

Sometimes melanoma is found in the skin, or just under the skin, but beyond a five-centimeter radius from the primary site. This special situation, referred to as *in-transit melanoma*, occurs when melanoma cells, trying to spread through the lymphatic vessels, get "stuck" and start to grow within the lymphatic vessels as a nodule just below or on the surface of the skin. Varying numbers of nodules may be anywhere between the primary site and the local lymph node basin. Seventy percent of in-transit melanoma cases are found on the legs and most of these patients have melanoma in the inguinal lymph nodes.

If the number of nodules is few and they are small in size, simple surgical excision can eradicate the melanoma; wide margins are not helpful. When there are many nodules or they are large, an *isolated limb perfusion* may be considered. Used exclusively for in-transit melanoma of the arms or legs, it's a procedure requiring the utmost technical expertise in both surgical and medical oncology as well as extensive equipment. High doses of chemotherapy are delivered to the affected extremity by isolating the blood flow into and out of the limb. The most commonly used chemotherapy agent is melphalan. Melphalan is derived from phenylalanine, an essential building block of melanin commonly found in melanoma cells. Melphalan, given in higher doses to an isolated extremity, appears to induce an anti-melanoma response. Interestingly this response can be even better when the extremity is warmed up to a temperature of about 41.5 degrees Celsius, a process called hyperthermia. This treatment results in complete disappearance of all melanoma in 50 percent of treated extremities and a partial response in 75 percent of patients.

The side effects of isolated limb perfusion include pain and swelling of the limb. The pain usually resolves in about two days and the swelling usually improves within two weeks.

In selected cases where surgical excision or limb perfusion is not possible, small in-transit melanoma nodules may be destroyed using a variety of techniques collectively referred to as *local ablation therapy*. A carbon dioxide laser has been very successful in removing small lesions, with few recurrences reported in early studies. Other experimental methods include photodynamic therapy, which destroys tumors by exposing them to high intensity light. Alternatively, bleomycin, a chemotherapy drug, can be injected along with electrical impulses directly into the lesions. In the past some lesions were successfully ablated by injection of live bacteria, such as BCG (Bacillus of Calmette and Geurin, used for tuberculosis prevention) and viruses, such as vaccinia virus (used for smallpox prevention). Any ablation therapy, because it is still experimental, requires caution and close monitoring.

Melanoma cells are somewhat sensitive to radiation; radiation therapy has been very useful for treatment, especially of large in-transit melanoma nodules. The radiation oncologist plans and administers radiation therapy. Outpatient treatment can often control in-transit melanoma in combination with other approaches.

Finally, in-transit melanoma may also be sensitive to other forms of *systemic therapy*, such as chemotherapy and immunotherapy. (See Chapter 8 for information.)

A FINAL WORD OF CAUTION

In-transit melanoma indicates the likelihood that the melanoma may have spread even further beyond the extremity. In fact, only 20 percent of patients with in-transit melanoma are alive five years after diagnosis. In-transit melanoma treatments can be challenging, and considerable judgment is required to select the most appropriate regimen. Treatment decisions should be made only after careful evaluation of the extent of melanoma spread to other sites in the body and discussion with an in-transit melanoma expert.

For many types of cancer, additional treatments may be used to decrease the chance of a recurrence and sometimes to prevent death from the cancer. Such treatment is referred to as *adjuvant therapy*. In the case of melanoma, adjuvant therapy is available but it does not provide as much benefit as for other types of cancer. (See Chapter 10 for more on adjuvant therapy.)

In situations where there is no effective therapy, patients can contribute important knowledge by agreeing to take part in clinical trials. If you are interested in participating in a clinical trial, read Chapter 15, which describes how to find the right one for you. Discuss this possibility with your physician, who may be able to help you find an appropriate study. Alternatively, you can search for clinical trials on your own using the resources listed in Appendix B.

Columbia Melanoma Center Case Studies

Marian is a sixty-year-old woman who noticed a mole on her right ankle was getting larger. A biopsy was done and an intermediate thickness melanoma was diagnosed. I performed a sentinel node biopsy and wide local excision of the melanoma on her ankle. The sentinel node I found in the right inguinal nodal basin contained melanoma. So I did a superficial inguinal lymph node dissection. Of the sixteen lymph nodes I removed, the only one with melanoma was the sentinel node. After an extensive discussion of adjuvant therapy, such as interferon-alpha, Marian decided against it.

Two years after her operation, Marian developed two small nodules on her calf about ten and fifteen centimeters from the primary ankle melanoma: in-transit melanoma. I surgically excised these two lesions without problems. A year later, she developed another in-transit melanoma lesion in the thigh, which I also surgically excised. Marian was well for another six years until she developed around fifteen nodules in the thigh and lateral knee of her right leg. She had no evidence of disease at any other site in her body and came to the Melanoma Center for consideration of isolated limb perfusion. During her pre-operative work-up, additional lymph node disease was discovered in the right inguinal and pelvic nodes. Marian agreed to enter a vaccine clinical trial and successfully completed the trial with no growth of her nodules. After the vaccine trial, one of her lower thigh lesions enlarged significantly to over fifteen centimeters. This area was treated with radiation therapy and the nodule slowly regressed and almost disappeared completely within three months. Marian then received systemic therapy with Interleukin-2 (IL-2) and has had a partial response in the nodules on her right leg.

Marian's is a complicated high-risk melanoma case diagnosed nine years ago. Although she refused interferon-alpha at that time, it is not known whether this would have delayed the time to recurrence of her disease. In the first few years she had relatively few nodules and they were small so simple surgical excision was appropriate. Once the disease progressed it became more difficult to control it. Surprisingly, she has not yet had melanoma spread to any internal organs although we continue to watch her carefully as she is at high risk for further disease progression. Marian represents an example of how expert clinical judgment and the combined use of surgery, vaccines, radiation therapy, and systemic therapy has led to the control of her disease for over nine years.

Ask Your Doctor

If you need treatment for melanoma in the lymph nodes, ask the following questions:

1. *Is a sentinel node biopsy indicated? How many of these procedures have you performed?* A sentinel node biopsy is indicated for all melanoma patients with a melanoma deeper than 1 millimeter in the skin. The procedure may also be indicated for melanomas greater than 0.75 millimeters but with other high risk features, such as ulceration, regression, male sex, young age, and location on the head, neck, or trunk of the body. Successful sentinel node biopsy requires skill; surgeons should perform at least ten to twenty procedures under supervision to attain adequate level of expertise. The sentinel node biopsy is best performed at the same time as the treatment of the primary melanoma.

2. *Do you use blue dye, radioactive tracer, or both?* Most surgical oncologists employ both radioactive tracers and blue dyes. Ask your surgeon about the complications of each. Lymphoscintigraphy greatly increases the ability of the surgeon to find the sentinel node and often allows for a smaller incision and more rapid operation.

3. *How does the pathologist evaluate the lymph nodes?* The pathologist checks for the presence of melanoma in the lymph nodes and, if melanoma is present, how many lymph nodes are involved. If stains for S100 and HMB-45 were also done, these immunostains increase the sensitivity of the pathologist's examination. A negative stain is very reassuring that melanoma has not spread. Likewise, some centers use polymerase chain reaction (PCR) analysis, which is more sensitive but has not been fully validated as a means of evaluating lymph nodes for melanoma cells.

4. *Do you use a drain after your node dissections?* If you are having a lymph node dissection, most surgeons use a drain to avoid complications after surgery. If your doctor is not planning to use a drain, you should definitely ask why not. I usually leave the drain in

for seven to ten days and allow patients to go home with the drain
after the nurses teach them how to take care of it at home. The drain
slips out easily in the office about a week later when the drainage
has decreased.

5. *What is your complication rate with this procedure?* Every surgeon
   should be able to quote you their complication rate for each
   procedure they perform. This information may also be available from
   your hospital or local health department. Just remember that every
   procedure has complications and rates below 10 percent are
   acceptable.

6. *Is adjuvant treatment available?* Once your operation is complete and
   the pathology report has been reviewed, you may be a candidate for
   adjuvant therapy. The reasons why you are or are not a candidate for
   additional therapy should be made clear.

7. *Is there a melanoma specialist available to discuss the treatment
   options?* Whether or not your surgeon feels you are a candidate for
   adjuvant therapy, you may want to talk to an expert in melanoma
   care. If your surgeon does not consider this his or her primary area
   of interest, ask for a referral. A serious discussion about the benefits
   and risks of high dose interferon, the only approved adjuvant
   therapy, should occur between you and your doctor. If you both
   agree that interferon therapy is appropriate, you should see a
   physician trained in the proper administration of interferon, typically
   a medical or surgical oncologist. If you decide that interferon is not
   appropriate for you, serious consideration should be given to
   participation in a clinical trial.

8. *What is the risk that the tumor has spread beyond the lymph nodes?* If
   melanoma is found in a lymph node you must ask about melanoma
   in other sites, especially elsewhere in the body. You will need special
   scans to make sure that the melanoma has not spread to distant
   sites, which would change the treatment plan. (See Chapter 9.)

CHAPTER EIGHT

How Do You Treat Metastatic Melanoma?

ONCE MELANOMA SPREADS to other parts of the body, a condition referred to as "metastatic melanoma," the average survival for most patients is between six and nine months. As frustrating and seemingly hopeless as such a diagnosis may be, an equal reality is that appropriate treatment and new experimental approaches are being tested continually. Over the years I have seen many people respond to treatment for up to several years, and even be cured of metastatic melanoma. One of the more puzzling questions in medicine is why some patients respond so well to therapy and others do not respond at all. Scientists are just beginning to understand the complex interplay between patient and cancer genetics and immune factors. Because occasionally we do see dramatic responses and cures for metastatic melanoma, it is vital for patients with metastatic melanoma to discuss their options with an expert and develop individualized treatment plans. Remember, if you don't respond to one type of therapy, you may respond to another.

General Approach to Metastatic Melanoma

Melanoma can metastasize—or spread—to almost any organ in the body, and the first thing I do when I see a patient with possible metastasis is determine exactly where the melanoma has spread. Knowing which body organs are involved and the extent of melanoma present are important factors to consider in recommending specific treatment options. Several tests that help define the location and amount of melanoma throughout the body are available, and I described them in Chapter 5 (see pages 95–98). The exact length of time for each of these tests varies, depending on the equipment and technicians available, but the range is usually between forty-five minutes and an hour. You may or may not be bothered by a sense of claustrophobia, mechanical noise, or having to lie still. If you are concerned about any of these possibilities, don't hesitate to ask your doctor to describe what you can expect in as much detail as possible beforehand.

In addition to the tests described in Chapter 5, a few other methods are used occasionally.

Arteriography is an imaging test in which special dyes are injected into an artery and X-ray pictures follow the arteries into specific body organs. While arteriography was helpful in the past to define tumors and normal anatomic structures, the use of CT scans has largely replaced this very invasive test. In difficult situations where there may be some question about a tumor or other abnormalities that are not clear from the CT scan, an arteriogram may be helpful.

A simple *chest X-ray* is a useful screening test for patients who are at lower risk for developing melanoma. If any abnormalities are found on a regular chest X-ray, then a CT scan should be obtained since this gives more information about the actual size of a tumor, its location, and its effect on the normal structures in and around the lungs.

Is there a blood test for melanoma? Routine blood tests may help to identify a problem but so far there is no absolutely proven blood test to find out if a patient has melanoma or if the melanoma has spread. A complete blood count to measure the number of white blood cells, red blood cells, and platelets may be useful as a general measure of health. Some patients with cancer will experience a decrease in their red blood cells and this may contribute to general feelings of fatigue and tiredness. The blood can also be tested for a number of enzymes the liver makes, which can sometimes be elevated when there is melanoma. One of these enzymes, the lactate dehydrogenase (or LDH), has been reported to be elevated in patients with very advanced melanomas. These tests should always be done, since patients with an elevated LDH blood test require immediate treatment.

Tests for Metastatic Melanoma

What tests should you have and when should they be done? There are actually very few studies to answer these important questions. Based on the few completed studies that have been done and my personal experience in taking care of melanoma patients for many years, I have developed a protocol for which tests we obtain. (See Table 8-1.) I want to stress that in specific cases the standard routine may change. The plan for testing must be individualized based on each patient's symptoms. For example, if a patient develops a severe headache, I would obtain an MRI of the brain immediately. If someone feels severe pain in the bones of the leg, I'd order a bone scan or plain X-ray of the bone, and so on.

**Table 8-1. The Melanoma Center's standard X-ray and
blood tests**

Stage of Melanoma	Imaging (X-ray) Tests	Blood Tests	Comments
I	None	None	The risk of spread is low; avoid sun exposure; routine skin examinations
II	Chest X-ray	Liver function studies, LDH	The risk of spread is small but patients should have these tests once a year

Stage of Melanoma	Imaging (X-ray) Tests	Blood Tests	Comments
III	Brain MRI; CT: chest, abdomen, and pelvis	Complete blood count, liver function studies, LDH	These tests are done as a baseline and every 3–6 months for 2 years and annually for another 3 years
IV	Brain MRI; CT: chest, abdomen, and pelvis; PET scan	Complete blood count, liver function studies, LDH	Studies every 3 months, PET scans in selected cases

Treatment Options for Metastatic Melanoma

I frequently tell my patients that this is a cunning disease, often complicated by setbacks and treatment failures. But just as often there are dramatic responses, and I believe that we must be aggressive about trying different treatments. Most of the time there is no way to predict which patients will respond to which treatments. I cannot overemphasize that we have many options for patients. Table 8-2 lists some of the treatment options available. An organized and logical plan for treatment is critically important. If one strategy is ineffective, then the next therapy should be ready to go. In addition, every patient should consider the many clinical trials available. (See Chapter 15.)

I also want to stress that treatment options must take into account your general health, any other medical problems, the chances for alleviating pain, and the quality of life that can be provided. Although my major goal is always to try to find a cure for my patients, sometimes I can't. In those cases, an equally important treatment goal is to help patients feel comfortable, suffer less, and support them in dealing with a terminal illness. This is the most difficult part of my job, and my team works hard to be realistic while providing appropriate hope for those patients who may be able to respond to treatment. I have many patients who have been able to beat the disease and remain alive and well more than ten years after being diagnosed with metastatic melanoma. They are a constant inspiration to me.

Table 8-2. General treatment plan for metastatic melanoma

Treatment	Benefits	Complications	Comments	Availability
Surgery	Offers best chance for cure	Similar to operations on involved part of the body	Best option for single lesions	Most comprehensive centers
Radiation	Provides immediate pain relief and may prevent recurrence at the site	Damages normal tissue and may lead to swelling and other problems	Treatment of choice for very large lesions or melanoma in the brain and bone not amenable to surgical removal	Most comprehensive centers
Chemotherapy	Provides immediate killing of melanoma cells	Many side effects are common; can damage the immune system	Useful when melanoma is growing rapidly; should be used after IL-2	Through most local oncologists
Immunotherapy	Can lead to long term responses and even cures	The side effects can be severe unless managed by an expert	The treatment of choice for most patients with more than one lesion and who can tolerate therapy	Selected comprehensive cancer centers

Treatment	Benefits	Complications	Comments	Availability
Clinical Trials	Provides access to new drugs and treatments	No guarantee of benefit, and side-effect profile often not established	Must be decided on an individual basis	Selected centers (see Chapter 15)
Re-staging Scans	New scans should be obtained after each treatment to determine the effects on the melanoma	Side effects of the additional radiation are small	Only scans can tell how well a treatment has worked; your doctor should obtain these at regular intervals*	Most medical centers

* A regular interval is usually every three months for patients with metastatic melanoma but may need to be obtained more frequently.

Surgery

If surgical removal of primary melanoma and lymph nodes is effective treatment for early stage melanoma, does surgical removal offer any advantage for metastatic melanoma? Surgical removal may be useful and can be life-saving in selected patients, depending on the number of melanoma lesions. When a single lesion is identified, surgery is the procedure of choice no matter where the melanoma has spread, including to the brain or any other internal organ. Surgery has been less effective, however, if there is more than one lesion, which is why it so important to identify melanoma lesions as early as possible. Approximately one third of patients who have successful surgery for a single melanoma lesion will be alive five years after their operation. Surgical removal of several sites of melanoma may also be contemplated following other treatments (such as immunotherapy), as there is mounting evidence that such combination treatment is helpful in selected patients.

The complications of the surgery will depend on where the melanoma has spread, but there are few locations that are not amenable to a surgical procedure. The surgery is best done by an expert in surgical oncology, preferably by a surgeon with melanoma experience. In addition, a neurosurgeon may be needed if the melanoma is in the brain whereas a gynecologic surgeon may be needed for metastatic melanoma involving the ovaries. The most important part of the operation is to make sure that all of the melanoma is removed. I often work with the appropriate specialist to make sure that all melanoma is removed at the time of the operation. My colleagues are usually happy to have the extra help, and such a multidisciplinary approach provides my patients with the best possible care.

Although successful operations that remove all melanoma place patients in a much more favorable position, they must still be followed closely. I obtain CT scans of the chest, abdomen, and pelvis as well as an MRI of the brain and blood tests every three months for the first two years after the operation. Following surgery, patients remain at very high risk for recurrent melanoma and may also want to consider a clinical trial testing new agents that are being tested to help prevent melanoma recurrence.

Chemotherapy

Over the last few decades a better understanding of how tumor cells grow and divide has provided new molecular targets for a host of new chemotherapy agents. The role of chemotherapy in melanoma, however, has been limited due to the relatively poor sensitivity of melanoma cells to most single-agent chemotherapy drugs. A combination of drugs improves the response to chemotherapy. Combination chemotherapy kills more cells since individual tumor cells may be resistant to one drug but vulnerable to another one. A disadvantage of combination chemotherapy is a higher rate of side effects, and so far no melanoma studies show that any particular combination of drugs prolongs the survival of melanoma patients compared to using a single chemotherapy agent.

The effectiveness of chemotherapy depends on the type of tumor, the number of tumor cells, the location of the tumor cells, the rate at which the cells are dividing, other molecular features of the tumor cells, and your general medical condition. While it may be possible in the near future to obtain a "profile" of all the genes and proteins in individual tumor cells to help guide which chemotherapy agents may be most effective, currently this is not possible. Therefore, the drug or drugs selected are based on large studies evaluating the response to chemotherapy in a group of patients with the same stage of melanoma. These studies have identified several specific chemotherapy drugs with some benefit against melanoma (see Table 8-3).

The effectiveness of specific agents is determined through clinical trials that study the drugs in various doses on patients with a similar type and extent of disease. Oncologists and pharmacologists have developed a set of objectives, called clinical endpoints, for these studies. If you hear your doctor say something like, "The response rate for this drug is 20 percent," he's referring to one type of clinical endpoint, the response rate, as opposed to another clinical endpoint, which could be the survival rate.

A response rate is a common endpoint of a clinical study and refers to whether the tumor responds to treatment at all. This is determined by measuring the size of all tumors before and after treatment with a particular drug. The measurement is usually done by a CT scan or similar imaging procedure. The National Cancer Institute has developed strict criteria for defining a response to treatment, and most investigators use these criteria when reporting the results of a drug study in melanoma. The most important response is called the *complete response*: the number of patients that have all of their tumor regress—or disappear—after treatment. A complete response also implies that no new tumors grew during treatment for at least four weeks. A complete response is distinguished from a *partial response*, which means that there was a 50 percent reduction in the amount of tumor in a patient without any new tumors forming. Another endpoint is *stable disease*, no change, or minimal change, in the tumor during treatment. Since most tumors grow over a four-to-eight-week period, stable disease may also be good news. You can begin to see the problem in being able to interpret your doctor when he says there is a 20 percent response rate. Ask your doctor if this is a 20 percent complete response rate, or overall response rate, which typically includes partial and sometimes stable disease responses as well.

Many studies also report survival data that is equally as important as (if not more important than) response rates. Although tumors may "respond" by shrinking, the effect may be short-lived, with tumors growing again very quickly after treatment stops. Survival statistics report how long patients live after treatment, and they may be reported as the percentage of patients who remain alive at a particular time marker, for example at one year. Alternatively, survival is sometimes reported as the average amount of time patients are alive after treatment. The *relapse-free survival* is the time that patients remain alive without evidence of tumor. If drug A has an average relapse-free survival of two years and drug B has a relapse-free survival of six months, we would choose to use drug A. Another commonly used endpoint is the *progression-free survival*, the amount of time patients are alive without tumor growth. Although a good measure of how effective drugs are at preventing tumor growth, it may not translate into actual tumor killing. Perhaps the most important endpoint for any drug study is the *overall survival*, the total amount of time patients live after receiving a drug. The only endpoint that demonstrates the ability of a drug to prolong life, this is the major endpoint usually accepted for FDA approval of cancer agents.

SINGLE AGENT CHEMOTHERAPY

A number of chemotherapy drugs have shown some benefit for metastatic melanoma patients. While overall response rates for these drugs are well defined, there is little evidence that any single agent prolongs survival in patients with metastatic melanoma. Still, many of these drugs can control the disease temporarily and alleviate symptoms associated with disease in what is referred to as palliative therapy.

While there are many other chemotherapy agents available, the following have received the most attention as possible drugs for melanoma patients. Your doctor may try other agents where there is less data available to document the effects on melanoma. New chemotherapy drugs are always being developed and may offer additional hope for melanoma treatment (see Chapters 12–14).

Table 8-3. Single agents used for the treatment of metastatic melanoma

Chemotherapy Agent	Response Rate (%)	Comments
Dacarbazine (DTIC)	15–20	Most commonly used single agent
Temozolamide (Temodar)	20	New oral DTIC analog that gets into the brain
Carmustine (BCNU)	10–20	Used mostly in combination regimens
Lomustine (CCNU)	10–20	Used mostly in combination regimens
Fotemustine	10–35	Used in Europe, especially for ocular melanoma
Vinblastine (Velban)	10–15	Used mostly in combination regimens
Vincristine (Oncovin)	10–15	Used mostly in combination regimens
Cisplatin (DDP)	15–20	Important agent used in many combinations
Paclitaxel (Taxol)	15–20	May be effective in some patients as single agent when others have failed
Docetaxel (Taxotere)	15–20	Similar to paclitaxel but fewer side effects

Dacarbazine (or DTIC) most likely works by altering the DNA and RNA in melanoma cells, making it difficult for the cells to grow and divide. DTIC is given intravenously and is usually administered once every three weeks in metastatic melanoma patients. The major side effect is a decrease in the white blood cell count and platelet count. Other side effects include nausea, vomiting, flulike syndromes for several days, and pain or burning at the site of injection. The nausea and vomiting can typically be prevented by using anti-nausea drugs before DTIC administration. Hair loss is not common with DTIC but the hair may thin out during treatment. DTIC has been the single most effective agent for melanoma, and nearly all studies comparing DTIC to other agents favor DTIC alone. The overall response rate is around 15–20 percent.

Temozolamide (or Temodar) is a relatively new analog of DTIC. Available as an oral pill, temozolamide is usually taken by mouth on an empty stomach at the same time every day. A typical schedule is five days in a row every twenty-eight days, but there are other regimens that have been used. Temozolamide gets converted in the liver to a smaller metabolite and can enter the brain and spinal cord, unusual for a chemotherapy drug. Temozolamide, already used for brain tumors, is being actively tested in melanoma and early studies have shown a slight improvement in survival with temozolamide compared to DTIC. The major side effects include bone marrow suppression (low white blood cell and platelet counts), nausea, and vomiting. An anti-nausea medication should be taken prior to temozolamide to help prevent this side effect. Other side effects include headache, fatigue, mild elevation of the liver enzymes, diarrhea, constipation, loss of appetite, and temporary change in taste, rash, and photosensitivity.

Carmustine (or BCNU) works by interfering with DNA, RNA, and protein synthesis in melanoma cells. Carmustine is given intravenously and also crosses into the brain, making it useful for treatment of brain melanoma. The response rates in melanoma have generally been much lower than those seen with DTIC or temozolamide so carmustine is most often used in combination with other chemotherapy drugs. The side effects are similar to those of DTIC. Additional side effects include damage to lung tissue, so you should tell your doctor if you develop shortness of breath or coughing after receiving carmustine.

Lomustine (CCNU) also interferes with the synthesis and function of DNA, RNA, and proteins in melanoma cells. Lomustine may result in cross-linking of DNA in melanoma cells, which prevents them from dividing properly. Lomustine is similar to carmustine except it is available in an oral pill form and is generally taken at bedtime on an empty stomach. The side effects include bone marrow suppression (low blood counts), nausea, vomiting, sore mouth, change in taste, loss of appetite, impotence, lung damage, kidney damage with high doses, neurologic damage, and increased risk of developing other types of cancer. Hair loss is not common.

Fotemustine has been tested in Europe for the treatment of ocular (eye) melanoma. Fotemustine was given by a pump implanted into the liver of patients with ocular melanoma that had spread to the liver. In this trial, sixty-two patients completed treatment and they reported an overall response rate of 35 percent with seven complete responses and fifteen partial responses. Another twenty-nine patients had stable disease and 27 percent of the patients survived for two years. The main side effects were bone marrow suppression (low white blood and platelet counts), elevation of the liver enzymes, nausea, vomiting, and abdominal pain. Further research is needed to see if fotemustine is better than the other agents.

Vinblastine (or Velban), an extract of the periwinkle plant, prevents microtubule formation in melanoma cells, which is required for the cell to divide. Vinblastine may also work by preventing DNA, RNA, and protein synthesis. The drug is given intravenously and has a low response rate in melanoma when used alone. The major side effects are temporary bone marrow suppression, nausea, vomiting, sore mouth, hair loss (usually reversible), high blood pressure, fatigue, constipation, diarrhea, peripheral neuropathy (numbness and tingling of the hands and feet), headache, fatigue, and pain at the tumor site.

Vincristine (or Oncovin) has a similar mechanism of action and response rate as vinblastine. Vincristine is given intravenously and the most common side effect is nerve damage. Constipation is also quite common and a good bowel regimen should be used to prevent severe constipation during treatment. Other side effects include abdominal pain, hair loss, skin rash, fever, bone marrow suppression, and hypersensitivity reactions.

Cisplatin (or DDP) binds to DNA resulting in a cross link of the DNA, which prevents the cells from dividing. Cisplatin is given intravenously and overall response rates in melanoma have been around 15–20 percent. The major sides effects include nerve damage (peripheral neuropathy), kidney damage, and bone marrow suppression (white blood cell, red blood cell, and platelet counts). Other side effects include nausea, vomiting, ear damage (hearing loss), loss of appetite, change in taste, elevation of liver enzymes, hair loss, and allergic reactions. Cisplatin is commonly used in combination regimens for patients with metastatic melanoma.

Paclitaxel (or Taxol) binds to the microtubules in melanoma cells to prevent cell division. Originally derived from the bark of the Pacific yew tree, paclitaxel is given by intravenous administration. The response rates for melanoma have been around 15–20 percent with a few complete responses reported. The side effects are temporary bone marrow suppression, hypersensitivity reactions (skin rash, flushing, redness, low blood pressure, shortness of breath), peripheral neuropathy (numbness and tingling of the feet and hands), low heart rate, sore mouth, diarrhea, elevation of the liver enzymes, fatigue, headache, abdominal and joint pains. Complete hair loss almost always occurs. Paclitaxel may be difficult to give to patients with diabetes, previous heart disease, patients with known liver damage, and those with preexisting neuropathy. Patients should also avoid sun exposure to the skin or nails after receiving six or more paclitaxel treatments. The use of steroids before treatment with paclitaxel may prevent the hypersensitivity reactions.

Docetaxel (or Taxotere) is derived from the needles of the European yew tree and works in a similar manner as paclitaxel. The response rates in melanoma patients are similar to paclitaxel as well. An advantage of docetaxel is a lower incidence of hypersensitivity reactions and neuropathy compared to treatment with paclitaxel. A fluid retention syndrome, characterized by weight gain, swelling, and fluid in the lungs or abdomen, sometimes occurs. Pre-treatment with steroids may prevent or reduce this side effect.

COMBINATION CHEMOTHERAPY TREATMENT

A single chemotherapy agent is rarely effective at completely eradicating established tumors. A combination of chemotherapy drugs has been a useful strategy for many types of cancer, such as leukemia, lymphoma, breast cancer, and colon cancer. Two popular regimens, listed in Table 8-4, are the M.D. Anderson and Dartmouth regimens, which have been extensively evaluated in clinical trials. The combination results in higher response rates compared to any single agent chemotherapy treatment. No benefit in overall survival has been demonstrated for these combinations, however. Side effects have been more severe when multiple agents are used, although the regimens in Table 8-4 have all been well tolerated by patients.

Response rate, relapse-free survival rate, and overall survival benefit, are what I consider when deciding on treatment for my patients. I like to develop a rational plan where we start with one type of treatment and move to another one if the first is not effective.

Patients with significant medical problems may not be able to tolerate certain chemotherapy agents. The chance of achieving a response needs to be balanced with the degree of probable side effects. The amount of disease and the rate of the tumor growth are also important features to consider. For example, when tumors are growing rapidly, the cells may be more sensitive to chemotherapy. Therefore, I often recommend chemotherapy when tumors are growing quickly, provided the patient can handle the drugs. We discuss the benefits of each agent and combinations of agents. Likewise we establish a sequence of chemotherapy regimens to use. I often suggest starting with a combination regimen if a patient is otherwise healthy since response rates are higher than single agents. If you don't respond to this treatment, one of the single agents can be considered. In patients with serious underlying medical illnesses we may elect to use single agent temozolamide rather than a combination regimen.

Table 8-4. Combination chemotherapy regimens for metastatic melanoma

Regimen	Chemotherapy Agents	Response Rate	Survival Benefit
M.D. Anderson	Dacarbazine (DTIC)	30–70%	No
	Vincristine (Oncovin)		
	Cisplatin (DDP)		
Dartmouth	Dacarbazine (DTIC)	40–50%	No
	Carmustine (BCNU)		
	Cisplatin (DDP)		
	Tamoxifen		

Radiation Therapy

Radiation is a form of energy and radiation therapy is a treatment that includes the use of both X-rays and gamma rays to kill melanoma cells. The mechanism by which radiation kills tumor cells is not entirely understood. While it is clear that radiation damages the DNA of tumor cells, which prevents the cells from growing and dividing normally, there is evidence that radiation has other anti-tumor effects. The local delivery of radiation releases a number of reactive molecules that may interfere with normal cell growth. Radiation also damages nearby blood vessels and may cut off the blood supply to tumors. More recently there

is evidence that radiation may help induce a local immune response to
fight cancer cells. Although this all sounds like a good way to eliminate
melanoma cells, the susceptibility of any individual melanoma cell to
radiation can vary. In addition, normal cells are also sensitive to the effects of radiation and so the benefits must be weighed against the risks
to normal cells.

Radiation is usually used for advanced cases of melanoma where
surgical removal is not possible and chemotherapy may be hard for
a patient to tolerate. Radiation therapy is the major method of treating melanoma in the brain and spinal cord. There is also new evidence emerging from research laboratories that radiation therapy
combined with immunotherapy may be especially effective. Radiation therapy needs to be carefully planned in coordination with other
treatment regimens. Even when it does not kill all the melanoma cells,
radiation therapy is especially useful as palliative treatment for reliev-
ing pain.

For those patients who may be candidates for radiation therapy, a radiation oncologist is consulted. A radiation oncologist is trained in the
use of radiation for the treatment of cancer. Many comprehensive medical centers have a department of radiation oncology where the radiation
oncologist has an office and access to the necessary machines. A number
of other radiation health specialists may be employed to coordinate
therapy for patients. Table 8-5 lists some of these specialists and their
role in planning radiation treatments.

Table 8-5. Radiation therapy health professionals

Health Professional	Job Description
Radiation oncologist	Physician trained in use of radiation for cancer therapy; acts as the primary doctor for radiation treatments
Radiation physicist	Scientist who plans complex treatments and performs all calculations of radiation dose and delivery

Health Professional	Job Description
Dosimetrist	Assists the scientist in calculating the radiation dose and planning the treatment schedule
Radiation therapy nurse	Licensed nurse who helps take care of patients undergoing radiation therapy
Radiation therapist	Technician trained in setting up radiation treatments and administering the therapy to patients

The amount of radiation used depends on the size of the tumor, the location of the tumor, the sensitivity of the tumor and surrounding normal tissues to radiation, and the type of radiation being used. Based on these considerations, a total dose will be calculated and then divided into smaller fractions to be delivered on different days. The number of days and schedule of treatment will then be determined. The radiation oncologist meets with the patient, discusses the process involved with the selected procedure, the side effects of radiation, and the treatment schedule planned. An imaging scan, such as a CT or MRI scan is typically used to locate the exact position of the tumor in the body. The body is often marked with a pen or similar device so that the tumor can be located during each radiation treatment visit.

Radiation may be delivered from an external source or from a source implanted inside the body. **External beam therapy** refers to radiation from an energy source outside of the body and uses a beam to direct the radiation to the tumor. The treatment usually lasts only a few minutes at a time. **Stereotactic radiosurgery** allows more accurate tumor targeting so that higher doses of radiation can be delivered while limiting the amount of damage to surrounding normal tissues. The procedure uses several powerful radiation beams at various angles that focus precisely on the tumor. **Gamma knife radiosurgery** is a specialized form of stereotactic radiosurgery and is especially helpful for the treatment of melanoma that has spread to the brain. The gamma knife technique is a non-invasive procedure that locates the melanoma by CT or MRI scan before the procedure. A lightweight frame is placed on the head using a local anesthetic before the MRI/CT scan. The radiation oncologist can localize the tumor site exactly and uses the head frame to precisely pinpoint the location of the melanoma. The "knife" is composed of 201 intersecting beams of radiation, resulting in a highly concentrated dose of radiation at the tumor site while avoiding normal brain tissue. It's similar to using a magnifying glass to concentrate the powerful rays of the sun in a single area. The procedure is completed on one visit but may require medication to prevent brain swelling and seizures. Gamma knife radiosurgery may be as effective as open surgical procedures, although it is best used on small melanoma lesions. In fact, some reports suggest that fewer than 10 percent of patients who have gamma knife radiosurgery have evidence of brain melanoma at the time of death.

Internal radiation therapy, also referred to as **brachytherapy,** is a procedure whereby radioactive material is placed inside the body to release the radiation at the site of a tumor. This approach, commonly used to treat prostate cancer, has not been as useful for melanoma. The high doses of radiation can damage normal cells if they are exposed to the radiation beam, which can lead to serious side effects. The most common side effect of radiation is fatigue, although other side effects depend on the exposure of normal tisues in the area of the radiation dose (see Table 8-6). It usually takes some recovery time after radiation treatments to feel better.

Table 8-6. Side effects of radiation therapy

Body Site	Side Effect
General	Fatigue, fevers, loss of appetite, increased risk of infection
Brain	Memory loss
Head and neck	Hair loss, sore or dry mouth, change in sense of taste and smell, difficulty swallowing

Body Site	Side Effect
Chest	Difficulty swallowing, chest pain, shortness of breath, cough
Abdomen	Loss of appetite, inability to eat, nausea, vomiting, abdominal pain, rectal bleeding, diarrhea
Skin	Redness, burning, loss of pigmentation

Immunotherapy

The immune system is a collection of cells and molecules that fight infections and disease. Nearly all types of cancer are somewhat susceptible to the immune system, but two types of cancer—melanoma and kidney cancer—are surprisingly vulnerable. Many strategies, referred to as "immunotherapy," use the immune system to destroy tumors. Immunotherapy differs from chemotherapy in a few important ways. Whereas chemotherapy destroys tumor cells immediately, immunotherapy needs time to activate immune cells and allow them to do their work. Chemotherapy can't distinguish between melanoma and other actively dividing cells, such as cells lining the gastrointestinal tract, which accounts for much of its severe side effects. Immunotherapy is capable of targeting only tumor cells and leaving normal cells alone. Many of the molecules on tumor cells are also found on at least some normal cells, so there still are side effects possible. In addition, if the immune system is overly activated, a severe disease called "autoimmunity" is possible. A major difference with immunotherapy is the ability of immunotherapy to cure a small but defined number of patients with metastic melanoma.

Immunologists have identified a number of new cell types and molecules over the last two decades and are beginning to understand how immune responses are generated. Exactly how the immune system fights cancer is not completely known. We know the immune system can fight cancer because there is evidence that cancer occurs at a higher rate in patients whose immune systems are impaired, such as people with HIV infection or transplant patients on medications that suppress the immune system. Additional evidence for the immune system's role in cancer is provided by the rare but well-defined episodes of spontaneous disappearance of cancer—most commonly reported with melanoma. Recently the immune system has been proven to detect and eliminate cancer as a normal function in animal models.

How Does the Immune System Fight Cancer?

The unique ability of the immune system to send out its soldiers as cells that can move throughout the body allows the elimination of an infection wherever it might occur. Highly specialized cells of the immune system, called lymphocytes, fight bacteria and viruses. Lymphocytes are part of the white blood cells. Broadly they contain two different kinds of cells—B cells and T cells. The B cells produce antibodies, molecules that attach to bacteria and target them for destruction by the immune system. Each B cell in the body makes one antibody that recognizes one bacterial protein. If the body is invaded by a particular bacterium, the immune system will activate the matching B cell to grow and divide, mounting an army of B cells to making antibodies against the bacteria. If enough antibodies are made, the bacteria will be defeated. If the bacteria can outgrow the antibodies, the infection can become serious and even threaten a patient's life. Fortunately, the immune system is very powerful and usually wins this battle. Once the infection is cleared, the immune response is shut off to protect the rest of the body from continued attacks. Importantly, some B cells survive to become *memory* B cells. These cells remain in the body, and if the person is invaded by the same bacteria again, the memory B cells mount an immediate attack and prevent the infection before it begins. This unique process is called immunity and protects us from subsequent infection by the same bacteria. Vaccines produce memory B cells, which is how vaccination protects us against many types of infection.

While B cells protect against bacteria, viruses are trickier to eliminate from the body. Lymphocytes primarily responsible for eliminating viruses are called T cells. T cells are found in similar places as B cells, but do not make antibodies. Viruses produce proteins that break down inside infected cells into small fragments called peptides. Peptides in turn bind to specialized molecules called HLA (human leukocyte antigen) complexes. T cells can identify peptides from viruses when they are bound to the HLA complexes. Once the T cell recognizes that a virus is present, the T cell can kill the infected cell, thereby eliminating the virus. This occurs through molecules released by the T cell that punch holes in the virus-infected cells and by signals to the infected cell programming the cell for a kind of suicide or cell death. Just like memory B cells, memory T cells are formed after a virus infection and protect against another infection by the same virus.

Another big piece of the immune response puzzle has recently been discovered: a type of white blood cell called a dendritic cell. These cells engulf—or eat—bacteria as well as virus-infected cells. The dendritic cells travel to the lymph nodes after encountering a bacteria or virus-infected cell and begin to signal both B cells and T cells to divide and attack the offending organism. After this activation process, which may cause swollen, painful lymph nodes, the lymphocytes travel back to the area of infection.

Recently, immunologists have also made the exciting discovery that dendritic cells can actually eat up cancer cells and work to activate T cells even more strongly. The fact that the dendritic cells in the skin are different from dendritic cells in other parts of the body may explain why melanoma is so susceptible to attack by the immune system.

Dendritic cells are important for another reason. Several types of T cells have slightly different functions. CD8+ T cells can fight infections (and probably cancer, too) by directly killing virus-infected or cancer cells. Sometimes we refer to these cells as killer T cells. In contrast, CD4+ T cells regulate immune responses and are called helper cells. Whereas CD8+ T cells can interact with many cells in the body, CD4+ T cells are activated only by specialized cells in the immune system, such as dendritic cells. Most experts agree that both CD4+ and CD8+ T cells are needed to fight a viral infection or cancer.

The cells of the immune system communicate with each other partly through molecules that are released into the circulation. Called cytokines, they influence the growth and survival of specific immune cells. Laboratories around the world are studying the effects of cytokines on the immune system. The interleukins are among the most well studied of the cytokines, and affect the interactions of the leukocytes (white blood cells). The CD4+ T cells are a major source of interleukins. Interleukin 2 causes T cells to grow, divide, and develop into killer cells that destroy virus-infected cells. Interleukin-4 has the same effect on B cells and is released during bacterial infections. To date, over 20 cytokines have been discovered and likely there are a few more. These cytokines play an important role in regulating immune responses.

We now believe that the immune system can recognize and destroy cancer cells in a similar manner to the way the immune system fights infection. Even less is known about how this occurs. Many immunologists think that the immune system may survey the body organs on a regular basis and eradicate small cancers when they arise. In cases where the cancer is small, the immune system may be able to eradicate the cancer. In situations where the immune system is weakened or there are too many cancer cells, the cancer may get out of control.

How the immune system recognizes cancer cells may be related to the most basic feature of cancer—the altered DNA causing protein mutations. Immunologists have identified a number of proteins—or antigens—in melanoma cells that can serve as targets for T cells. These antigens are also under investigation as targets for vaccines. In addition to mutated proteins, some proteins are produced in large quantities by melanoma cells as compared to normal melanocytes. The large number of proteins may lead to their preferential delivery to the HLA molecules and they may be able to attract T cells.

*   *   *

YOU WILL SEE in Chapter 13 how this information is being used to develop vaccines against melanoma. Surprisingly, one of the best treatments for melanoma has been one of the cytokines involved in regulating T cell responses, namely interleukin-2.

Interleukin-2

To date, the most effective immunotherapy for melanoma and kidney cancer has been interleukin-2, or IL-2 for short. IL-2 is a cytokine that promotes the survival, growth, and killer functions of T cells. IL-2 is normally produced by the immune system in very small quantities. In the late 1970s, researchers using recombinant DNA technology were able to produce large amounts of IL-2. This revolutionized the field of immunology in several ways. First, efforts to study T cells in the laboratory had proven difficult since most T cells do not survive for long outside the body. If they are exposed to IL-2, however, they continue to grow and can survive for long periods of time. Thus, IL-2 was essential in helping immunologists to study T cells in the laboratory. Perhaps even more important, IL-2 activates T cells in the body and has been effective in treating some forms of cancer, most notably metastatic melanoma and kidney cancer. IL-2 is being evaluated for its effects on other cancers as well.

The amazing thing about IL-2 is that some patients respond so well that all the melanoma may be destroyed. In fact, a small number of patients (around 5–10 percent) will have a complete response to IL-2 and may even be cured of metastatic melanoma. An additional 10–15 percent of patients will have a partial response to IL-2 treatment. Perhaps the most intriguing thing about IL-2 is that those patients who develop any type of response often go into remission for three to four years! Clearly better than any type of chemotherapy, such success led to the FDA approval of IL-2 for kidney cancer in 1992 and for metastatic melanoma in 1998. *At the present time IL-2 is the single best treatment for metastatic melanoma.*

IL-2 has been most effective in high doses, typically around 600,000 units per kilogram. Lower doses of IL-2 have been used but should only be used as part of an experimental regimen. The lower doses are often used with vaccines, for example, to boost the level of immune response. The safest way to give IL-2 is to have patients in a medical setting where the heart rate, blood pressure, and urine output can be measured efficiently. The average hospitalization lasts about five days. A liquid preparation, IL-2 is given intravenously every eight hours. Patients should receive as many doses as possible up to a total of fifteen doses. There is often about a day or so for recovery until patients can go home. I allow a two or three week interval and then repeat another week of IL-2. Once two full cycles have been given to patients, a CT scan or similar test is done to evaluate the effects of the IL-2 on the melanoma. If the melanoma is responding, we can repeat the IL-2 until all disease disappears. If there is no response, then we move on to another treatment.

We cannot predict who will or won't respond to IL-2 treatment. In general, patients who are in better overall medical condition and those patients who are able to tolerate a large amount of IL-2 tend to do better. I have, however, seen patients with very large melanomas receive only a few doses of IL-2 and have a complete disappearance of all melanoma.

The best way to prevent complications from IL-2 is to make sure that patients have no significant risk factors before starting treatment. Patients should also avoid any type of steroid medications, such as prednisone or Decadron, since steroids counteract the effects of IL-2. The major side effect is low blood pressure, so IL-2 may stress the hearts of patients with heart disease. All patients over the age of fifty or those with heart disease should have a stress test before receiving IL-2. These tests may be physical, as in walking on a treadmill, but the heart's ability to withstand stress can also be tested by administering certain drugs that cause a more rapid heartbeat. Another common side effect is an accumulation of fluid, which can lead to swollen arms and legs, or swelling of internal organs. The brain is especially sensitive to even a small amount of swelling so an MRI scan of the brain is essential. IL-2 can also make autoimmune diseases worse, especially ulcerative colitis and thyroid disease, so IL-2 may not be possible in patients with these disorders. The most serious side effect is infection, which can be prevented with antibiotics.

The good news is that most of the side effects associated with IL-2 can be prevented with pre-medication. More good news is that nearly all of the side effects with IL-2 are reversible; they resolve once the treatment is stopped. In fact, most side effects clear up within a few days. Nonetheless, patients receiving IL-2 need to be monitored very closely and IL-2 should only be given in a hospital setting with personnel who have appropriate monitoring experience.

Table 8-7. IL-2 side effects and treatment

System	Side Effects	Treatment
Whole body	Fever and chills	Tylenol and Indocin before each dose
	Itchy skin	Eucerin cream or medications (Benadryl, Atarax)
	Weight gain	Diuretic medications (Lasix)
Brain	Confusion	Stop IL-2
	Hallucinations	Stop IL-2
Heart	Low blood pressure	Fluid administration or medications to raise the blood pressure
	Abnormal heart rhythms	Stop IL-2 and medications (Digoxin)
Lungs	Shortness of breath	Medication (Lasix) or oxygen; rarely draining fluid by a needle or mechanical assistance for breathing

System	Side Effects	Treatment
Blood	Low platelets Low red blood cells Low white blood cell count	Reverses on its own Blood transfusion Reverses on its own; antibiotics
Liver	Elevation of liver enzymes	Reverses on its own
Kidney	Elevated creatinine	Reverses on its own; close monitoring of kidney function
Endocrine	Low thyroid function	Thyroid medication
Gastrointestinal tract	Sore mouth Nausea and vomiting Diarrhea	Lidocaine mouthwash Anti-nausea medication Medications (Immodium)
Immune system	Infection Autoimmunity	Antibiotics Stop IL-2 or steroids in severe cases

Developing a Treatment Plan

I hope that by now you see that there are actually quite a few treatment options for melanoma, including surgery, chemotherapy, radiation therapy, and immunotherapy. If these treatments fail, you can consider entering into a clinical trial, which is covered in Chapter 15.

How do you decide which treatment to use? By consulting a doctor experienced in treating melanoma patients to help you develop a plan.

Let me explain why a plan is so important. If there is a single lesion—no matter where in the body it is located—surgical removal offers the best chance for a cure. This holds true even if the melanoma has spread to the brain. As most chemotherapy does not enter the brain, time spent trying it may reduce the chances of a cure or long-term survival. Or, if a patient's melanoma does not respond to chemotherapy, IL-2 may not be as effective because the immune system may be damaged by the chemotherapy itself. Therefore, in those patients who can tolerate high dose IL-2, I generally prefer to try that first and save chemotherapy for later, if necessary.

That said, I know of no definitive rules for making a treatment plan. In Table 8-2 I list some general strategies that will help you to discuss a treatment plan with your doctor—if possible, a doctor who specializes in the treatment of metastatic melanoma. Many resources are available to help you decide on treatment options.

Columbia Melanoma Center Case Studies

Henry was twenty-seven years old when he noticed a black mole on his left leg begin to grow. He went to his dermatologist, who performed a biopsy and revealed a malignant melanoma that was 2.5 millimeters deep. He had a wide local excision by his local surgeon and recovered well. Three years later he developed a nodule in the left groin and a biopsy revealed melanoma in the lymph nodes. His surgeon performed a lymph node dissection to remove all of his lymph nodes from the left groin. He also opted to have interferon-alpha therapy for one year after his operation. Four months after stopping interferon, however, he noticed a lump on his chest and a biopsy confirmed that it was metastatic melanoma. Since this was a single melanoma and no other disease could be found anywhere else in his body, he underwent surgery to remove the lump.

He was well for another two years, when he developed severe stomach cramps and distention. A CT scan showed extensive melanoma in his abdomen blocking his small intestines. He was evaluated by a surgeon, who removed the blocked small bowel but was unable to remove all of the melanoma from the abdomen. His local oncologist gave Henry chemotherapy with dacarbazine (DTIC). His melanoma did not respond and was growing in his abdomen.

When I first met Henry at the Melanoma Center, he was very anxious and complained about his abdomen feeling bloated and crampy. He had no history of heart disease, autoimmune disease, or any other serious medical problems. His scans showed that there was no melanoma in his brain or lungs, but a large amount of melanoma could be seen throughout his abdomen lining the outside of the intestines. We decided to try IL-2, since he had not had immunotherapy and was in good health other than his melanoma. Henry tolerated the IL-2 quite well and after the first two cycles he began to feel better. A repeat CT scan showed the melanoma was shrinking, so we continued to give him more IL-2. After another two cycles the melanoma continued to shrink until only two small areas remained. We stopped the IL-2 and decided to wait and see what would happen with these two areas of disease. Both areas remained about the same size for almost one year, but a PET scan showed activity in both areas, suggesting that live melanoma cells were still present. We therefore decided to operate on Henry to see if we could remove these areas. He underwent surgery. We successfully removed two melanoma tumors and saw that the remainder of his abdomen looked normal. Henry recovered nicely and had no complications from his operation.

Although Henry, now thirty-five years old, appeared to have no evidence of melanoma, he was worried about his risk of the melanoma recurring. Henry was asked to participate in a clinical trial testing a new peptide vaccine designed to prevent melanoma from recurring after surgical removal. He agreed to participate in the clinical trial and was able to receive a series of vaccinations. Henry has now been free of his melanoma for four years and is back at work leading a full and productive life.

Henry represents a true success story and is a good example of how careful treatment planning is important for patients with metastatic melanoma. He was quite frustrated in the beginning, since so many treatments, including surgery, interferon, and chemotherapy, did not seem to be beneficial. Careful planning and close follow-up medical care provided other options that appear to have been much more helpful for this patient. The combination of high dose IL-2 and surgical intervention gave Henry four years of melanoma-free life. In addition, he may be receiving additional protection from his participation in a vaccine clinical trial. When I first met him,

Henry had a prognosis of only six months. I have now known him for nearly five years and often ask Henry to talk to other patients with metastatic melanoma, as he is an example of how successful treatment can be even in the face of a poor prognosis.

Ask Your Doctor

If you need treatment for metastic melanoma, ask the following questions:

1. *Why do you recommend this particular treatment?* When developing a treatment plan with your doctor you should ask why he or she recommends a particular plan. You should also ask what they will do next if this treatment is not successful, not only for your peace of mind but also because some treatments may prevent subsequent treatments. For example, chemotherapy may weaken the immune system and not allow IL-2 treatment. Likewise, some clinical trials may not allow prior therapy with specific agents, so you should know what clinical trials might be available to you. For example, if there is a small melanoma lesion in the brain, radiation therapy or surgical removal may be required before other treatment can be considered. It is important to distinguish between reasons that relate to your medical condition from reasons related to what is available at your doctor's practice site. It is not unusual for patients with difficult disease, like metastatic melanoma, to be referred to other doctors or centers for treatment. You should be comfortable that your doctor is thinking about your best interests.

2. *Do you offer IL-2? Why not?* High dose IL-2 is not offered in all hospitals yet may be helpful for many patients with metastatic melanoma. If your doctor does not offer this treatment, you should ask if she or he knows someone who does offer IL-2. If your doctor does not know, you can find a center close to you by consulting Appendix A at the end of this book, which lists centers across the United States that treat melanoma patients with high dose IL-2.

3. *Am I a candidate for a surgical procedure?* Since the best chance for a cure is currently with surgical removal it is important to be

absolutely certain whether an operation is feasible. Your doctor should be able to determine if this is a reasonable option and refer you to a specialist in melanoma surgery.

4. *Am I a candidate for a clinical trial?* Always ask what clinical trials are available through your doctor or hospital. In general, the larger the hospital the more likely there will be a clinical trial available. See Chapter 15 for more details.

5. *How often will I have CT scans during or after treatment?* The effectiveness of any given treatment can only be truly measured by CT or MRI scans. Therefore you should ask about how often these will be obtained. It is also important to have a scan just before starting any treatment as a baseline. Typical intervals are about every two to three months for scans.

6. *What are the response rates for the various treatment options?* As you consider each option, take into account the success of the treatment, the side effects of the treatment, and whether a treatment will exclude you from other treatments later. Remember there is a difference between response rate and survival so you need to ask about both. Treatments that provide better survival are always better than those with good response rates. The side effects should also be carefully considered when developing a treatment plan, since time is needed for recovery from any type of treatment.

CHAPTER NINE

How Do You Treat Melanoma in Special Sites or Situations?

S O FAR I'VE focused on cutaneous melanoma, which accounts for 85–90 percent of all melanoma. Some patients, however, develop melanoma in a site other than the skin. The most common sites are the eye (ocular melanoma) and the mucous membranes (mucosal melanoma) that line the mouth, nasal cavity, sinuses, and the anus. Other atypical melanoma sites are the brain and the fingers, toes, and under the nails.

These melanomas behave in a slightly different manner than cutaneous melanomas. In this chapter, I discuss these rare variants and how treatment differs from cutaneous melanoma.

Patients with melanoma who do not have a skin melanoma and who have never noticed an abnormal mole or skin melanoma should have their eyes examined carefully by an ophthalmologist (a doctor specializing in diseases of the eye). In addition, a careful examination of the mouth, throat, nasal cavity, and sinuses should be performed. A rectal examination should also be done and can be easily accomplished in the office setting by a trained physician.

Patients with melanomas at special sites are often excluded from participating in melanoma clinical trials, so less information is available about the efficacy of various treatments. This does not necessarily mean that therapy will not work, but rather that we do not know as much about how such patients respond to therapy.

In addition to special sites, melanoma may occur in some unexpected segments of the population. For example, melanoma may occur in children—I recently saw a seven-year-old boy with cutaneous melanoma and an eight-year-old girl with ocular melanoma. Reports of melanoma in pregnant women suggest that this form of melanoma may be particularly challenging to treat. These special patients require additional thought and expertise in developing a treatment plan.

Melanoma in the Eye (Ocular Melanoma)

Ocular melanoma represents 70 percent of all cancer affecting the eyes. Ocular melanoma is divided further into uveal and conjunctival melanoma (see Figure 9-1). Uveal melanoma can appear in the iris, the choroid, or the ciliary body. Conjunctival melanoma occurs in the conjunctiva.

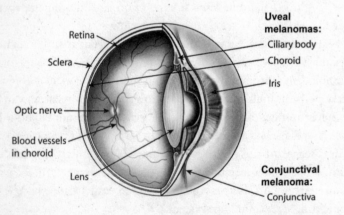

Figure 9-1. Anatomy of the eye and location of typical ocular melanomas

Most ocular melanomas show up in the uvea with only 2 percent arising from the conjunctiva. In many cases it is not clear exactly where in the eye the melanoma started. The risk factors are similar to those for cutaneous melanoma, with some evidence of a genetic cause. The specific genes involved have not been identified. Sun exposure, especially ultraviolet radiation, is a probable risk factor. In addition, patients with the dysplastic nevus syndrome and nevi or freckles of the eye may be at increased risk for developing ocular melanoma, making frequent eye examinations for patients with known dysplastic nevus syndrome essential. A link between ocular melanoma and other types of cancer, including breast cancer, ovarian cancer, lymphoma, and melanoma of the skin, has been reported.

The risk of ocular melanoma increases with age, but the disease does occur occasionally in children. Ocular melanoma is more common in Caucasian populations, and while it affects both genders equally, there may be a trend toward occurring in younger females and older males. As in many forms of cancer, early treatment leads to high cure rates. Survival after metastatic disease is typically only two to five months, so early detection and treatment is important.

Symptoms and signs vary depending on the melanoma's location and size. Sometimes it is a small irregular mole on the outer parts of the eye. A larger melanoma may lead to glaucoma, visual changes, or pain. Any new symptoms should be investigated by an eye specialist or ophthalmologist.

Pathologists can identify two major types of ocular melanoma cells. Spindle cells have an elongated or spiny shape or appear as small and round. In contrast, epithelioid cells are larger and more likely to be dividing. Spindle cell melanomas tend to mean a better prognosis, whereas epithelioid melanomas are worse. Occasionally, melanomas have mixed spindle and epithelioid cells.

Because there are no lymphatic vessels in the eye, ocular melanoma does not spread to the lymph nodes. Rather, these melanomas spread through the blood and most commonly go to the liver. While ocular melanoma can spread to nearly every organ, almost 100 percent of patients with metastatic ocular melanoma have melanoma in the liver. A CT or MRI scan of the liver should be obtained for any patient with a large ocular melanoma.

In ocular melanoma a careful ophthalmologic examination, not a biopsy, is used for the diagnosis. The ophthalmologist looks into the eye after dilating the pupil in a procedure called **indirect ophthalmoscopy.** Sometimes additional techniques are helpful. Scleral transillumination, in which light is directed against the white part of the eyes, can sometimes show a melanoma provided that it has pigment. Another technique, especially for distinguishing a melanoma from a hemorrhage (small area of bleeding), is videoangiography. In videoangiography an imaging tool takes pictures of the eye after a dye has been injected into the small blood vessels. Melanoma lesions have a characteristic appearance that can be seen with a scanning laser or similar imaging device. Ultrasound is another imaging system, especially useful for large melanomas. The ultrasound can define the exact size of the melanoma and determine if it is attached to surrounding structures. Color-coded Doppler ultrasound may also provide information about the blood flow into the melanoma. In difficult cases a fine needle aspiration biopsy can be considered. In this procedure a tiny needle is inserted into the nodule and a small number of cells are extracted.

Several factors influence how we treat ocular melanoma. Most important is the size of the melanoma. Size is difficult to calculate for ocular melanomas since we do not biopsy and measure the melanoma. Instead, two traits help determine the true size of an ocular melanoma. Most ocular melanomas assume a dome-shaped configuration (see Figure 9-2). The apical height of the melanoma, or the maximum height the melanoma extends from its base, and the diameter of the dome's base can be determined through the ophthalmoscope or through ultrasound examination. Ocular melanomas are classified as small, medium, or large, based on the apical height and diameter of the base as described (see Table 9-1). A fourth category, diffuse, is assigned to those rare melanomas that are not dome-shaped.

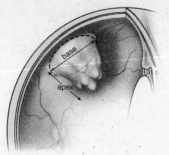

Figure 9-2. Typical nodular or dome-like appearance of an ocular melanoma. The height of the dome and diameter of the base determine the size classification (see Table 9-1).

Table 9-1. Classification of ocular melanomas

Classification	Apical Height	Largest Basal Diameter
Small	1–3 millimeters	5 millimeters
Medium	2–10 millimeters	16 millimeters
Large	> 10 millimeters	> 16 millimeters
Diffuse	<20 percent of the basal dimension	Horizontal or flat pattern

The treatment for ocular melanoma depends on the size classification, the location in the eye, and whether the melanoma has spread into nearby structures around the eye or to other organs.

A major issue is the ability to preserve vision for patients whenever possible. In situations where vision is already compromised by the melanoma or the effects of melanoma on the eye, such as the development of severe glaucoma, it may be best to remove the eye. This may also be true for melanomas that are very close to the optic nerve and when conservative treatments may result in loss of vision. These are difficult decisions to make and referral to an expert in ocular melanoma is recommended.

Melanoma of the Iris

The iris is the colored portion of the outer eye that surrounds the pupil. Similar to the aperture of a camera, the iris controls how much light enters the eye. Small muscle fibers in the iris dilate or widen the pupil when it is dark and constrict or narrow the pupil when exposed to light. The color of the eye, unique for every person, is due to melanin produced by melanocytes within the iris. The main risk factors for melanoma of the iris are exposure to sunlight and certain genetic alterations.

Both melanoma and benign nevi can develop in the iris. Photographs help to follow the lesion and determine the effects of treatment. Overall, the outcomes for melanomas of the iris are good, with 95 percent of patients alive five years after diagnosis. The cells are usually the spindle type, which also has a better prognosis. Therefore, conservative treatment—simple observation—is possible. However, surgical removal of the eye may be necessary if the melanoma begins to grow quickly or if it is already very large.

Most patients naturally find contemplating eye removal very distressing. While it is perfectly understandable to recoil at the idea, the procedure itself is straightforward and patients do just fine.

Eye **enucleation,** which is a total removal of the eye, can be very effective treatment for melanoma. It's also quite rare: Enucleation is not performed as frequently as in the past because other effective treatments are available. For very large melanomas, however, situations where the melanoma is causing severe glaucoma, or when the melanoma is attached to structures outside of the eye, enucleation may be necessary. If the eye is removed, obviously vision will be lost, although most patients should be able to see well from the other eye. About six weeks after surgery a prosthetic eye can be fitted by an ocularist.

In an alternative to eye enucleation, only the melanoma is removed, leaving the eye intact. Called **local resection,** this procedure can be used for medium-size melanomas (see Table 9-2). Although it may seem like the best option, significant risks of complications are associated with local resection. The complications can include bleeding into the eyeball (vitreous hemorrhage). Retinal detachment, where the retina is disrupted, can occur. Proliferative vitreoretinopathy is a severe scarring reaction that involves the retina. These conditions can affect vision and so the outcomes may be no better than that of enucleation.

Another option is called plaque radiotherapy, which is a form of local radiation treatment. The "plaque" refers to a round gold cap that is placed over the melanoma in an operation. A radioactive seed is placed under the cap to focus the radiation on the melanoma. Because the radiation cannot escape from the gold cap, the remainder of the eye and body are protected. The surgery is usually performed in the operating room and patients must stay in the hospital for four or five days. The cap is then removed in another short operation. The plaque radiotherapy technique protects the body and non-exposed parts of the eye; however, vision can be affected by damage to the parts of the eye under the gold cap, including the retina and optic nerve. The success of plaque radiotherapy may be improved by using an ultrasound to guide the exact placement of the gold cap at the time of the operation, and many centers are now routinely using ultrasound for this purpose.

Table 9-2. Treatment options for melanoma of the iris

Size	Treatment Option	Comments
Small	Observation	Must be no symptoms; close follow-up with photography is required

Size	Treatment Option	Comments
Medium	Local resection	Surgical procedure; useful if melanoma is growing rapidly
Large	Enucleation	Removal of the entire eye; necessary if the melanoma is very large, causes severe glaucoma, or spreads outside the eye
	Plaque radiotherapy	Non-invasive alternative to eye removal surgery

Melanoma of the Ciliary Body

The ciliary body, a small structure located just behind the iris, contains numerous small fibers that attach to the lens of the eye. These fibers change the shape of the lens, which alters the ability to focus on objects close by or far away, a process called accommodation. The ciliary body also produces a clear fluid called aqueous humor that fills the front part of the eye. Melanoma of the ciliary body is rare but can be very serious, since it is often found late and has a worse prognosis than melanoma of the iris. This may be related to the difficulty in making the diagnosis, since melanoma of the ciliary body mimics many other more common diseases of the eye (like glaucoma and chronic uveitis). Several options for treating ciliary body melanoma are listed in Table 9-3.

In addition to the treatment options mentioned for iris melanoma, the use of external-beam, charged-particle radiotherapy has been used for ciliary body melanomas. This procedure uses a precisely focused beam of radiation from an external machine. The procedure requires a patient capable of fixing the eye on a single point (where the radiation beam is coming from) for a prolonged period of time. The technique uses sophisticated equipment that is only available at specialized centers. The rate of complication is higher with external-beam treatment.

Table 9-3. Treatment options for melanoma of the ciliary body

Treatment Option	Comments
Plaque radiotherapy	Procedure of choice for small lesions; high incidence of cataracts as a complication
External-beam, charged particle radiotherapy	Available only in specialized centers; may be as effective as plaque radiotherapy but complication rate is higher
Local resection	Useful for small, thick lesions
Enucleation	Procedure of choice for large melanomas

Melanoma of the Choroid

The choroid is located between the sclera (the "whites" of the eye) and the retina in the back of the eye, where the optic nerve transmits images to the brain. The choroid contains layers of blood vessels that provide nourishment to the back of the eye. This is a common area for ocular melanomas to develop.

The diagnosis of choroidal melanoma can be very difficult, since there are often few symptoms when the melanoma is small. Any choroidal lesion that exhibits growth over time should be highly suspicious for melanoma. Choroidal melanoma treatment has been highly controversial (Table 9-4). In the past, many ophthalmologists thought that observation alone was acceptable for small melanomas, since there was little evidence that therapy protecting the eye was possible. New research suggests that treatment of small melanomas of the choroid do improve the survival rate for patients. Large melanomas of the choroid can have a very poor prognosis and often require eye enucleation for control. Therefore, there has been a steady trend toward earlier treatment for all choroidal melanomas.

Table 9-4. Treatment options for melanoma of the choroid

Treatment Option	Comments	Indications
Observation	Consider when diagnosis uncertain, no tumor growth is documented, or in elderly and debilitated patients	Small lesions only
Plaque radiotherapy	Similar to plaque radiotherapy for other ocular melanomas	Small and medium lesions
External-beam, charged-particle radiotherapy	Similar technique as for other ocular melanomas; melanoma must not be located near the optic nerve	Small lesions
Gamma knife radiosurgery	Similar technique as used for melanoma in the brain	Small lesions
Laser photocoagulation	Uses laser directed through an ophthalmoscope; may be combined with plaque radiotherapy	Small lesions
Transpupillary thermotherapy	Uses heat to destroy tumors; may be combined with plaque radiotherapy	Small lesions
Local resection	Similar to local resection for other ocular melanomas	Small lesions with greater thickness
Enucleation	Procedure of choice for large lesions; should be used in all cases where vision cannot be saved	Large lesions or medium lesions with extensive melanoma
Combined therapy	Useful for larger lesions and typically combines plaque radiotherapy with another method	Medium and large lesions

Conjuctival Melanoma

The conjunctiva is a thin, transparent layer of tissue that covers the sclera and lining of the inside of the eyelids. The conjunctiva secretes small quantities of oils to lubricate the eye. Although a rare event, the conjunctiva can develop melanoma. It often appears as a pigmented black growth, making it easy to spot. When the melanoma is in the intermediate layers, it can be difficult to detect except by a trained ophthalmologist who can look into the pupil.

Melanoma in the Mucous Membranes

The membranes that line the inner layers of the digestive and respiratory tracts contain mucous, which is secreted to help aid digestion and help remove small particles from the breathing passages. These mucous membranes include melanocytes, hence melanoma can develop. Mucosal melanoma is quite different from melanoma of the skin. It often is very difficult to diagnose because it mimics other diseases. Even an experienced physician can mistake it for something else. Mucosal melanomas have a particularly poor prognosis, although why they are so aggressive is not known.

Mucosal melanomas may occur in the mucosal lining of the nose, mouth, upper respiratory tract, and sinuses. Symptoms depend on exactly where the melanoma is located and how big it is. Common symptoms include headaches, nasal stuffiness and runny nose, difficulty swallowing or breathing, wheezing, cough, and occasionally coughing up blood or blood tinged mucous. You see that these symptoms are similar to the common cold, sinusitis, asthma, bronchitis, and many other conditions. If these symptoms persist despite other treatments, a search for an underlying tumor should be done.

The diagnosis is made by careful examination of the lining of the nose, sinuses, upper respiratory tract, and throat. An otorhinolaryngologist, otherwise known as an ear, nose, and throat (or ENT) doctor, uses an instrument with a tiny camera to visualize the mucosal lining. If he sees something abnormal, he can perform a biopsy through the inserted scope to confirm a mucosal melanoma. These melanomas may also show up on a CT scan or MRI but the scans only show a mass and cannot provide a definite diagnosis. The only way to be sure of a melanoma, whether cutaneous or mucosal, is by examining tissue under a microscope.

The cause of mucosal melanoma is not known, although some evidence suggests that sun exposure may be a factor. Genetics may also be involved. This type of melanoma has not been studied that well by scientists, in part because it is so uncommon.

The first thing is to consider before deciding on treatment is whether the melanoma is truly a mucosal melanoma. Melanoma from the skin can metastasize to the mucosal linings. A primary skin melanoma can hide in hard to see places, such as under the scalp, behind the ears, and on the back. Sometimes the skin melanoma regresses, or disappears, probably because the immune system attacks the melanoma in the skin.

If there is no primary skin melanoma, the melanoma may have originated in the mucosal membrane. In this case, making sure there is no spread from the site is important. Imaging or scans of the brain, chest, abdomen, and pelvis by a CT or MRI scan is necessary because mucosal melanomas can metastasize to almost any other internal organ and they do so more frequently than skin melanomas.

Mucosal melanomas that have already spread should be treated like metastasized skin melanoma (see Chapter 8). Most treatments have not been as effective for mucosal melanoma, as they are for skin melanomas. Many clinical trials do not include patients with mucosal melanomas because they are known to be less responsive to treatment. Patients do occasionally respond and so it is always worth trying some form of therapy. I have used high dose IL-2 for many patients with mucosal melanoma and several patients have responded. Chemotherapy has been less successful but may delay the growth of some mucosal melanomas.

In mucosal melanomas that have not spread there may be a chance for cure. Treatment options include surgical resection and radiation therapy. The decision must be individualized based on the location and size of the melanoma. For small melanomas that are easily reached by the surgeon, a surgical resection is the best choice. Radiation can reduce the size of larger melanomas and relieve pain.

In most cases mucosal melanomas represent diagnostic and therapeutic challenges for patients and their physicians. We commonly use multiple treatments for our patients with mucosal melanoma and the timing of surgery, radiation, and systemic therapy needs to be logically planned and delivered.

Melanoma in the Anus

Melanoma in or around the anus is referred to as anal melanoma. These melanomas may grow in the skin just outside the anus, the anus itself, or in the mucosal lining of the rectum, similar to mucosal melanomas in the head and neck region. Anal melanomas tend to be very aggressive and are frequently difficult to diagnose. The treatment options for anal melanoma are also controversial and differ from the treatments that we recommend for melanomas of the skin.

Most of the time anal melanoma is misdiagnosed. Many patients may be treated for hemorrhoids instead of anal melanoma, as a common symptom for both is minor bleeding from the rectum, especially just after going to the bathroom. Other symptoms include anal pain or pain during bowel movements, itchiness, change in bowel habits, and unexplained weight loss. Physical examination may reveal a small mass inside the anal canal or extending outside of the anus. If a suspected hemorrhoid does not respond quickly to hemorrhoidal treatments, your doctor should consider a biopsy or removal of the hemorrhoid. Occasionally an anal melanoma is found incidentally after removing a hemorrhoid. Anal melanoma may or may not have pigment so the color of the mass is not helpful in making the diagnosis.

Anal melanomas are slightly more common in women and tend to be found between the ages of fifty and sixty, although they can occur in younger or older patients as well. The cause of anal melanoma is not known but may be similar to other types of melanoma.

The prognosis for anal melanoma is much worse than for melanomas of the skin. Anal melanomas can spread to lymph nodes in the groin region as well as to lymph nodes deep in the abdomen. In addition, anal melanoma can spread to internal organs, including the lungs, liver, and bone—it is not unusual to find anal melanomas spreading to almost any body organ.

The agreed upon treatment for anal melanoma is surgical removal but the extent of the operation is controversial. In the past a procedure called an **abdominoperineal resection** was commonly performed. This operation removes the entire anus and a portion of the rectum. With a significant risk for post-operative complications, the operation also condemns patients to a colostomy for the rest of their lives. This might be acceptable if the operation cured patients or improved their survival; little proof exists that this is the case. Many experts now question the wisdom of using an abdominoperineal resection for patients with anal melanoma.

Local resection in which only the melanoma and a small portion of surrounding tissue are removed is a better option, especially for small anal melanomas. It can be done through the anal opening and there is no need for a colostomy in most cases. The complications are fewer than with abdominoperineal resection and recovery is faster. Studies suggest that patients treated by local resection actually have a better outcome, but these may be misleading, since the two procedures have not been directly compared and it may be that local resection has been used more commonly for smaller melanomas.

At the Melanoma Center, we prefer to perform local resection for small or intermediate melanoma lesions. This is nearly always possible. All patients undergo a complete work-up to make sure the melanoma has not spread before any operation is considered. If lymph nodes are involved with melanoma but the rest of the body is clear, a lymph node dissection will also be performed. Our anal melanoma patients with mestastatic disease have derived some benefit from high dose IL-2 treatment and they should be offered IL-2 or chemotherapy. Until we have well designed studies to fully evaluate these treatment options for anal melanoma, we cannot fully know how effective these treatments will be.

Melanoma in the Brain

The spread of cutaneous or other melanomas to the brain is one of the worst possible situations since survival is limited and melanoma in the brain can lead to neurologic symptoms. The symptoms depend on where the melanoma is in the brain, the number of melanoma lesions present, and how rapidly they are growing. Symptoms may include severe unrelenting headaches, changes in vision, difficulty in speaking, memory lapses, vomiting, or numbness and weakness of the arms and legs. I usually order an MRI of the brain on all melanoma patients with Stage IV disease, and if any of these symptoms occur, I order an immediate MRI.

Although the prognosis is poor once melanoma has spread to the brain, aggressive treatment can prolong life. Table 9-5 lists some of the treatment options, which depend on how many melanoma lesions are present and their exact location. In patients with a single melanoma lesion, surgical removal (craniotomy) is usually the first step. This often relieves symptoms and patients live longer. The neurosurgeon must be able to remove the melanoma without disrupting normal brain tissue, however. Thus, early consultation with a neurosurgeon is necessary to determine if a patient is a candidate for a craniotomy.

Most patients with large brain metastases from melanoma benefit from steroid medications such as Decadron and prednisone. Steroids decrease the amount of swelling in the brain and often improve symptoms dramatically. A disadvantage is that steroids can inhibit the immune system, a problem for patients who are receiving or contemplating any form of immunotherapy. The side effects of steroids include stomach irritation, which can lead to peptic ulcers. The stomach should be protected with an antacid or other anti-ulcer medication. Other side effects include weight gain, fluid retention, abnormal chemistry balance, muscle weakness, osteoporosis, delayed wound healing, increased appetite, and worsening of diabetes. Fortunately, most patients only require steroids for a brief period of time.

Another very effective way to treat melanoma in the brain is with radiation therapy. The gamma knife radiation treatment, described in Chapter 8, is preferred for small, easy-to-reach metastases. The gamma knife can be used on multiple lesions in one procedure, and most patients can go home the same day. Side effects have been few but include seizures, typically occurring in patients with a history of a seizure disorder, and swelling, which can be treated with a short course of steroids. The gamma knife improves survival: More and more patients are alive one year after gamma knife radiation, especially if the brain was the only site of melanoma. The gamma knife procedure can be repeated if melanoma recurs in the brain, although the total amount of radiation that can be given to any one area is limited.

In patients who have many melanoma lesions (more than four) or very large melanoma lesions (larger than three centimeters) the gamma knife procedure may not be as effective. In these cases whole brain radiation can be considered. The use of whole brain radiation is complicated by the need to give high doses of radiation to kill melanoma cells and the sensitivity of normal brain tissue to radiation. Permanent complications include memory loss and confusion. The use of whole brain radiation following surgery or gamma knife procedures is controversial. I would probably only consider whole brain radiation in patients who have had multiple recurrences in the brain. But this decision must be considered carefully for each individual patient.

The use of chemotherapy in patients with brain metastases from melanoma has gained new popularity since the introduction of temozolamide (Temodar). This particular agent, which comes in an oral pill form, can actually enter into the brain and can kill melanoma cells. Early studies have suggested that Temodar is helpful for the treatment of melanoma in the brain. Further studies are necessary to know exactly how effective this therapy will be. Nonetheless for patients with brain metastases the use of Temodar should be considered.

Immunotherapy may offer some hope to patients with melanoma in the brain. In a study evaluating patients who had surgery for brain melanoma, patients who had received immunotherapy and had some response to the treatment before surgery survived much longer than patients who did not respond to the same immunotherapy. More recently, I have treated patients with gamma knife radiation and, provided there is no swelling, I begin IL-2 treatment. Patients have had remarkably few side effects from either the radiation or IL-2. Many have lived more than one year and remain well.

I trust that this discussion has convinced you that there is some hope for patients with melanoma in the brain. If you want to explore every option, find a specialist in treating patients with melanoma invading the brain.

Table 9-5. Treatment options for melanoma in the brain

Treatment Modality	Treatment Option	Comments
Surgery	Craniotomy	Procedure of choice for single lesions; performed by neurosurgeons with definite benefit for most patients
Radiation	Gamma knife	Helpful for multiple, small lesions; can be repeated
	Whole brain radiation	Unproven benefit; may be useful for many, large melanoma lesions
Medications	Steroids	Relieves symptoms; short course is preferred
Chemotherapy	Temozolamide (Temodar)	This agent crosses into the brain and kills melanoma cells
Immunotherapy	Interleukin-2 (IL-2)	May improve survival if given after treatment of brain lesions with surgery or radiation therapy

Melanoma of the Fingers, Toes, and Nails

Melanoma on the fingers, toes, and nails is rare and accounts for fewer than 2 percent of all cases of melanoma. These melanomas can have a worse prognosis than melanomas that occur on the other areas of the arms and legs. Melanoma that occurs under the nails is called **subungual melanoma.** These are especially aggressive and are often not diagnosed until late. They can be confused with fungal infection of the nails, which is much more common, or nail hemorrhage, bleeding under the nail. Hemorrhage may occur with trauma, such as when you slam a door on the tip of your fingernail or bang your toes on the edge of the bed. However, these should clear up in one or two weeks. If there is no traumatic event or if nail changes do not improve quickly a biopsy should be performed to make sure it is not a subungual melanoma. The most commonly affected sites are the thumb and great toe. Subungual melanoma may occur more frequently in African American individuals for reasons that are not known.

Unlike melanomas of the skin, subungual melanomas are aggressive no matter what their thickness. Therefore, all subungual melanomas should be treated by an amputation of the affected finger or toe. A sentinel node biopsy should also be performed to make sure that the melanoma has not spread to the lymph nodes. I want to stress the importance of having an amputation for these subungual melanomas. I have known patients who have tried to have a more limited procedure. All of them developed metastatic melanoma and none of them survived. Therefore amputation, although it may sound harsh, is an essential part of the treatment. The good news is that the amputation can be limited. If you look at your finger, you will see there are three segments with a joint in between each one. The appropriate amputation for most subungual melanomas is what we call a distal amputation, removing only the third of the finger at the end containing the nail. This leaves little functional impairment. For toes, the entire toe is removed but this is tolerated remarkably well. A metastatic work-up should be done if the sentinel node is found to contain melanoma. If the lymph nodes contain melanoma, a lymph node dissection at the location of the sentinel node is necessary. Adjuvant therapy should also be considered if the melanoma has spread to the lymph nodes.

Melanoma in Children

We may think of melanoma as a disease of adults, but we are diagnosing melanoma more frequently in children under the age of twenty. Some reports have found that children have thicker melanomas at diagnosis compared to adults, but this may be because melanoma is not generally considered in children and it takes longer to make the diagnosis.

While moles are common in children, any child who has a large number of moles, moles that have changed their appearance, or those children with a close relative who has had melanoma, should be evaluated by a dermatologist. Any suspicious moles should have a biopsy as we would recommend for adults. A Spitz nevus is a type of mole that has features very similar to melanoma. Spitz nevi are often found in children and can be difficult to distinguish from a true melanoma. (For additional information on how to recognize spitz nevi, see page 17.) There is an increasing trend for some pathologists to consider these two diagnoses as a continuum with the Spitz nevus being more benign and the melanoma being more serious. In any event, if there is any doubt at all the lesion should be treated as if it is a melanoma.

The treatment of melanoma in children is similar to that for adults. At present, it appears that melanoma behaves in a similar manner with response to treatment and prognosis related to melanoma thickness and presence of metastasis. Therefore, children should be treated in a manner similar to adults. We have treated children with high-dose IL-2 at our center without any significant complications. Therefore, most children should be considered candidates for IL-2 and other treatment regimens that have proven effective in adult melanoma patients.

Once melanoma is found, a child must be followed to make certain that there is no recurrence. Regular imaging scans and blood tests based on the stage of melanoma at diagnosis are part of the suggested follow-up for children listed in Table 9-6. The amount of radiation exposure, although small, is more substantial for children. Weigh that fact against the risk of melanoma recurrence and metastasis, which can be fatal if allowed to progress. Patients should have regular scans, chest X-rays, and blood tests for two years and then annually for another three years. The risk of recurrence decreases beyond five years, but patients should be examined by a qualified doctor at least once a year indefinitely.

Genetics may play a stronger role in childhood melanoma. Still, sun exposure should be minimized as all children who have had melanoma are at high risk for developing melanoma throughout their lives. The same precautions used in adults should apply to children. This includes avoiding excessive exposure to sun, using protective clothing and hats when sun exposure is possible, and wearing sunscreen with an SPF of at least 30.

Family members of a child with melanoma are also at increased risk of developing melanoma: Parents, brothers, and sisters should be screened and monitored carefully.

Table 9-6. Recommended follow-up for children with melanoma

Stage of Melanoma	Follow-Up Test	How Often?
Early stage (thin melanomas)	Skin examinations; keep out of the sun	Once a year
Intermediate stage (thicker melanomas)	Chest X-ray, blood tests (liver enzymes, LDH)	Once a year
Advanced stage (spread to lymph nodes or other organs)	Brain MRI; CT: chest, abdomen, and pelvis; blood tests (liver enzymes, LDH)	Every 6 months for first 2 years and then annually for Stage III disease; every 3 months for metastatic disease

Melanoma in Pregnancy

We used to think that melanoma was more aggressive when it occurred during pregnancy. Recent reports suggest that this is not the case. Melanoma behaves the same in pregnant women as it does in any patient. Pregnant women may simply have a diagnosis later than most other adults, since melanoma is so unexpected. Any pregnant woman who has signs of a melanoma, such as a change in her moles or a new pigmented lesion, should see her doctor immediately. A biopsy has almost no risk to the pregnancy and can be done to make sure that the mole is not a melanoma. When a melanoma is found the management can be difficult and depends on the stage of both the melanoma and the pregnancy.

If a melanoma is discovered in the first trimester of a pregnancy, a biopsy should be performed. If the melanoma is thin, treatment is a wide local excision and this can be safely performed using a local anesthetic. If the melanoma is more advanced and may have spread to the lymph nodes or internal organs, treatment decisions become more complicated. However, the health of the mother is important for the health of the fetus and so treatment should not be delayed. Ultrasound can compensate for CT scans, especially in the abdomen and pelvis, so that radiation to the lower abdomen can be avoided. There have been rare reports of melanoma spreading into the fetus and, although this is an extremely rare occurrence, it also speaks for the importance of treating the melanoma. In rare cases where the disease is quite advanced, the pregnancy may need to be terminated. Many of the systemic treatments, including chemotherapy and immunotherapy, are not safe for a fetus and cannot be administered to pregnant women.

If the melanoma is discovered during the second trimester, it should still be treated by initial biopsy to make the diagnosis and wide local excision can be performed for early stage melanomas. If the melanoma is advanced, a metastatic work-up should be done as well. Treatment decisions must be made in consultation with the obstetrician, pediatrician, and melanoma specialist. These decisions can be very difficult and require individual management as every case is different and requires a different approach.

Melanoma found in the third trimester is easier to deal with since the fetus is at lower risk of complications and the woman may be able to deliver before starting systemic treatment. Nevertheless, a coordinated plan should be developed. A biopsy and initial treatment are indicated, but further adjuvant or systemic therapy can usually be safely delayed until after delivery. An early induced labor may be useful to expedite melanoma treatment provided the fetus is able to survive.

Although melanoma during pregnancy can be devastating news, early and individualized treatment can save the life of both mother and child. This is a special situation where expertise in the management of melanoma is essential for developing a rational treatment plan.

Columbia Melanoma Center Case Studies

Ellie is a thirty-eight-year-old woman who developed mild rectal bleeding after her bowel movements. Her primary care doctor diagnosed hemorrhoids and gave her stool softeners and instructions for warm baths. After several months of this conservative treatment, she was not feeling better and had had episodes of pain. She underwent a hemorrhoidectomy, an operation to remove the hemorrhoids. The pathologist examining the hemorrhoidal tissue found an anal melanoma in the specimen. Ellie was then referred to a surgeon who recommended an extensive operation called an abdominoperineal resection, which removed the entire end of the rectum and anus. She agreed to the operation, handled the surgery without complications, and became used to having a colostomy.

Approximately one month after her operation, a CT scan of Ellie's chest and abdomen revealed a tumor in her liver. A biopsy confirmed that the tumor was metastatic melanoma. She was told that there was no effective treatment and that she had less than six months to live. Ellie and her husband came to the center for a second opinion.

I decided to treat Ellie with high-dose IL-2, since chemotherapy has not been effective for anal melanoma. She began treatment, which she tolerated quite well. After one course of treatment a new CT scan showed that the melanoma had shrunk to about half its original size. She was treated again with IL-2 and the disease went into remission for more than two years. During a routine visit two years later, I found a small lymph node in her neck, and a CT scan identified new melanoma lesions in her lungs. We discussed several options and decided to try a new vaccine that was being tested in a clinical trial. Ellie received three vaccinations with no side effects. Three months after entering the vaccine study a repeat CT scan showed that her disease was stable. She continued to do well for another six months.

During her next visit I noticed that the lymph node in her neck had started to grow again. I removed the lymph node and treated her with radiation to the neck after the operation. Ellie recovered well and continued to be stable for another year.

One year after completing the radiation to her neck I detected an increase in the melanoma in her lungs and also a new melanoma lesion in her adrenal gland. We decided to give chemotherapy a try this time as few other options remained. She tolerated the chemotherapy and continued to feel well for another six months. Ultimately, though, the melanoma progressed and she died four years after diagnosis.

Ellie represents a good reason to try various treatment options. A large operation, like an abdominoperineal resection, may not have been the best plan and should only have been done after determining that the melanoma had not spread. The decision to treat her with IL-2 and vaccine proved useful, as she did survive for more than four years with metastatic disease. This is especially good for patients with metastatic anal melanoma, and such patients should be encouraged to seek treatment whenever possible.

Ask Your Doctor

If you need treatment for melanoma in a special site or situation, ask the following questions:

MUCOSAL AND ANAL MELANOMA

1. *Is the melanoma a primary mucosal melanoma or metastatic from the skin?* While melanomas arise in the mucous membranes it is actually more common to have a skin melanoma spread to the mucous membranes. Your doctor should perform a careful examination to make sure that there is no other source for the melanoma on the skin.

2. *What treatment options should be considered?* The treatment options for early stage, small mucosal melanomas include surgical removal, which should be considered whenever possible. Radiation is also good treatment, especially for those mucosal melanomas in locations not easily reached by the surgeon. If the melanoma is more advanced or large in size you may need additional treatment. This must be individualized and discussed with an expert in caring for patients with mucosal melanomas.

3. *Should I have an abdominoperineal or local resection?* For anal melanomas the decision to have a large operation or a more limited local operation should also be individualized. The decision depends on how big the melanoma is at diagnosis and the presence or absence of metastatic disease. You may want to discuss this with an expert in melanoma before committing to a big operation. The trend has been toward more limited surgical removal and earlier institution of adjuvant therapy.

SUBUNGUAL MELANOMA

1. *Do I need to have a sentinel node biopsy?* The only treatment for subungual melanoma is amputation of the end of the finger or an entire toe. Most patients should probably also have sentinel node biopsy if there is no evidence of metastatic disease. Subungual melanoma does not depend on the thickness, so treatment is amputation, metastatic evaluation, and sentinel node biopsy if the metastatic work-up is normal.

2. *How often should I have scans?* Patients with subungual melanomas should be followed closely, since over half will develop metastatic

melanoma in the lymph nodes or internal organs. Your doctor should develop a logical plan for you after treatment is completed.

MELANOMA IN THE BRAIN

1. *How many melanoma lesions are there?* Among the most important features of melanoma in the brain is how many lesions are present. If only one lesion is present, treatment should consist of surgical removal if possible.

2. *How large are the melanoma lesions?* Another factor to be considered is the size of the melanoma lesions. Melanoma that is less than three centimeters responds well to localized radiation treatment, whereas larger lesions may not respond.

3. *Where is the melanoma located?* The success of surgery or radiation depends in part on where the melanoma is located. Melanomas that are close to the surface of the brain are easier to remove at the time of the operation than those located deep in the brain. Likewise, some parts of the brain are involved with important body functions, such as breathing, vision, and movement. Surgical or radiation treatment to these areas may have more serious side effects than when dealing with melanoma in a part of the brain with non-important body functions.

4. *What treatment options are available here?* If you are not at a major tertiary medical center there may only be a few limited options for treatment. It is necessary to know whether the expertise for dealing with melanoma in the brain exists at your center. Treatment planning and implementation require many experts, including neurosurgeons, radiation oncologists, and medical oncologists with experience in melanoma.

5. *Are there other options available at other centers?* Melanoma in the brain is among the most serious clinical conditions, and you should consider all possible options. Find out if a gamma knife radiation machine is available at a nearby center if it is not available at your hospital. Your doctor should be able to refer you to an excellent center with appropriate physician experience and equipment for treatment.

. *What systemic therapy should I have after the brain is treated?* Once melanoma is found in the brain it takes precedence over the treatment of melanoma at other sites. The brain should generally be treated first, since most people will die of their brain disease before succumbing to melanoma in other locations. Therefore, everything else is typically stopped so that the brain can be treated. However, once the brain is treated with either surgical or radiation therapy, attention should be turned to the rest of the body. Temozolamide is an excellent chemotherapy since it enters the brain tissue, and may also treats melanoma at other body sites. We have started to use high-dose IL-2 with some success in selected patients when the brain lesions are completely eradicated by surgery or radiation therapy.

MELANOMA IN SPECIAL POPULATIONS

1. *What is the treatment plan?* The diagnosis of melanoma in children, pregnant women, and other special populations requires treatment plans to be developed in consultation with experts in melanoma. Your doctor may be able to help with many of the tests and procedures required but should consult with an expert in melanoma to make sure that appropriate management and follow-up are provided.
2. *What is the plan for follow-up care?* No matter how old the patient, once a melanoma is identified, lifelong care is needed. This should be clear to the patient, his family, and his personal physician.
3. *Should other family members be tested?* The diagnosis of melanoma in young children suggests the possibility of strong genetic factors. This may place close relatives at risk for developing a melanoma. Therefore, relatives may want to speak with a genetic counselor about genetic testing. All relatives should see a dermatologist for annual skin examinations, learn self-examination by reading this book or from another source, and seek medical attention early if they develop any signs of melanoma.

CHAPTER TEN

What Should You Do After Treatment for Melanoma?

Once your treatment is completed, no matter what stage of disease you had, living with melanoma will require ongoing care. This chapter examines what "ongoing care" means and how to protect yourself from a recurrence of melanoma.

In patients who have had one melanoma the risk of a second melanoma is nine hundred times higher than the risk for a person with no previous melanoma. Although there is no foolproof way to prevent a second melanoma, the single best advice I have is to check your skin regularly for signs of a new melanoma. The monthly skin self-examination described in Chapter 3 and an annual professional skin examination are the best methods for detecting melanomas when they are still small and manageable.

The use of sunscreen with an SPF of 30 or 45 is probably worthwhile, although the effects of sunscreen in preventing melanoma are still uncertain. Sunscreen does help prevent other types of skin cancer and skin damage in general, so it seems sensible to recommend sunscreen if you must be out in the sun. My better advice is to avoid sun exposure if at all possible. This includes wearing protective clothing—long sleeve shirts and pants, hats to cover the scalp and face, and umbrellas or other protection if outdoors for prolonged periods. Do not even consider sunbathing or tanning salons, which are very high-risk activities that are known to promote melanoma formation.

Follow-Up Care for Stage I Melanoma

If you have a Stage I melanoma you should feel relatively comforted to know that most of these will not recur. Stage I melanoma virtually never spreads to lymph nodes or internal organs. Therefore surveillance of internal organs is not necessary. However, living with a Stage I melanoma does require careful skin examination and avoiding sun exposure. Do monitor the skin everywhere on your body for a second melanoma. Local recurrence, the development of a new melanoma within five centimeters (or two inches) of a previously removed melanoma, is also possible.

Table 10-1 lists the recommended timetable for skin care after treatment.

Although the risk of metastasis is low, it is not zero. Any new lumps or swollen glands should prompt an immediate visit to the doctor and a biopsy. Similarly, any unusual symptoms should be investigated. Remember, even in the face of metastasis, the earlier you seek treatment, the better your chance for a positive outcome.

Table 10-1. Follow-up recommendations for Stage I melanoma patients

Recommendation	How Often?
Avoid sun exposure; use sunscreen	Daily
Self skin examination	Once a month
Professional skin screening	Once or twice a year
Seek medical help for new lump or symptoms	As needed

Follow-Up Care for Stage II Melanoma

Stage II melanomas are generally curable, but the risk of recurrence or spread is higher than that for Stage I melanomas. Therefore, patients with Stage II melanoma should be monitored a bit more closely. Relatively few studies have evaluated the effectiveness of screening procedures, such as blood tests or body imaging scans. Nonetheless, careful attention should be paid to any new lumps, moles, or other unusual symptoms. The recommended schedule for follow-up care is in Table 10-2.

In addition to avoiding sun exposure and having routine self and professional skin examinations, two additional tests may help catch a recurrence. A simple chest X-ray can sometimes detect small abnormalities in the lungs. If a chest X-ray is not normal, a CT scan should be obtained to confirm the findings. It is not unusual to have some small nodules show up on a chest X-ray, especially in older people. This is normal and a CT of the chest can help to document the benign nature of these nodules and to know what "normal" nodules a patient has. In the future a repeat CT scan of the chest can be compared to a baseline scan. This is often helpful to distinguish a melanoma from a benign condition. I sometimes will get a CT scan just to have as a baseline scan for those patients with high risk Stage II melanomas.

While a validated blood test does not exist for the diagnosis of melanoma, other valuable information can be obtained through routine blood tests. The liver is a common site of metastatic spread, and when the liver is filled with melanoma (or any other tumor) the liver enzymes in the blood may become elevated. This can be detected by a routine blood test. The lactate dehydrogenase, or LDH level, correlates with advanced melanoma. Yet often many hospitals and laboratories don't measure LDH levels, as it has not been useful for diagnosis of liver disease. However, the LDH is important in following melanoma patients. If the LDH or other liver enzymes are elevated, I do a full evaluation of the body for sites of melanoma recurrence. An MRI of the brain and a CT scan of the chest, abdomen, and pelvis are routinely obtained at our center for any patients with an elevated LDH.

Table 10-2. Follow-up recommendations for Stage II
melanoma patients

Recommendation	How Often?
Avoid sun exposure; use sunscreen	Daily
Self skin examination	Once a month
Professional skin screening	Twice a year
Chest X-ray	Once a year
Liver enzymes, LDH blood test	Once a year
Baseline CT scan for very high risk patients	Once
Seek medical help for new lump or symptoms	As needed

Follow-Up Care for Stage III Melanoma

Patients with Stage III melanoma require much closer surveillance and follow-up than the Stage I or II patients. Nearly half of patients with Stage III melanoma will have the melanoma recur, most likely as metastatic disease. Since we cannot yet predict where the melanoma will recur, all potential areas should be considered and evaluated on a regular basis.

The skin should be examined carefully, as for any patient with a previous melanoma. The same recommendations to avoid sun exposure are valid for Stage III patients. Melanoma can return in the same lymph node basin if the dissection was not complete and even sometimes when the operation removes all of the lymph nodes. Patients should be examined by a doctor who can sometimes feel new lumps in the area of a previous operation.

Detecting metastatic disease is the main concern for Stage III patients, and I use an aggressive follow-up plan for at least five years to find new melanoma sites as quickly as possible. The good news is that if melanoma does recur it usually does so early. About 80 percent of patients who will develop metastatic melanoma do so within the first two years after the lymph node dissection. Nearly all patients will have a recurrence within five years. If the melanoma has not returned in that time, I switch back to the recommendations for Stage II melanoma patients (Table 10-2). Although the risk for recurrence is much less after five years, I have seen patients develop recurrences up to fifteen and even twenty years later. Thus, some follow-up is necessary for life.

In addition to routine self and professional skin examination for Stage III patients, I obtain a CT scan of the chest, abdomen, and pelvis every three months for the first two years (see Table 10-3). For the next three years, scans are every six months. An MRI of the brain every six months for two years and then once a year for the next three years is also recommended. Blood tests to include the liver enzymes and LDH are done every six months during the first five years after treatment. If you remain free of disease for five years, the recommendations for Stage II melanoma patients are fine.

In place of the MRI and CT scans, a PET scan is an acceptable screening scan. As discussed in Chapter 8, PET scans are very sensitive for melanomas but only when they are greater than 1–2 centimeters in size. An advantage of PET scan is the ability to image the entire body with one scan. You and your doctor can discuss the benefits and risks of each test. An important point is to be sure to use the same test for follow-up. The results are better when you use the same machine, since each type has minor differences in the quality of the images and ability to define the tissue. The radiologist will always compare the current films to previous scans when available. It also is important to return to the same radiologist to maximize the benefit of follow-up scans for detecting melanoma early.

Table 10-3. Follow-up recommendations for Stage III melanoma patients

Recommendation	How Often?
Avoid sun exposure; use sunscreen	Daily
Self skin examination	Once a month
CT scan chest, abdomen, and pelvis	Every 3 months for 2 years, then every 6 months for 3 years, then as needed
PET scan	As an alternative to CT or MRI, every 3 months for 2 years, then every 6 months for 3 years, then as needed
Brain MRI	Every 6 months for 2 years, then once a year for 3 years, then as needed
Liver enzymes, LDH blood test	Every 6 months
Professional skin screening	Twice a year
Seek medical help for new lump or symptoms	As needed

Adjuvant Therapy for Stage III Melanoma

Patients with Stage III melanoma may benefit from adjuvant therapy, treatment to prevent a recurrence of melanoma in high-risk patients. Stage III patients are definitely high risk.

The only United States Food and Drug Administration (FDA) approved adjuvant treatment for melanoma is an immune agent called interferon-alpha. The interferons are a group of proteins made by a variety of cells in the body. Interferon proteins are produced in response to viral infections and are called interferons because they work to "interfere" with virus production. Studies show the most effective interferon protein for melanoma is interferon-alpha. Interferon-alpha can directly kill melanoma cells in the laboratory. In addition, interferon-alpha can stimulate the immune response resulting in an attack on melanoma cells. Interferon-alpha also blocks blood vessels feeding tumors. Scientists do not entirely understand which of these mechanisms is the most significant for treating melanoma despite a large number of clinical studies evaluating interferon over the last twenty years. Although there continues to be great controversy over the results of these studies by experts in the field, considerable evidence suggests that interferon-alpha is effective in selected situations. Side effects can be significant, but they can be safely managed by experienced physicians and should not preclude interferon administration in appropriate patients. Nonetheless we know that the benefits of interferon are modest at best and clearly better treatment options are necessary.

Radiation therapy may offer protection against a recurrence of melanoma, especially at sites of lymph node involvement, at least in selected cases. In situations where there are many lymph nodes, or in which melanoma has spread outside the lymph nodes, radiation also may be helpful, especially for melanomas of the neck and axillary nodal basins. The decision to use radiation therapy requires consultation with the radiation oncologist and a melanoma specialist. The amount of radiation used depends on the size of the nodal basin and the extent of disease at the time of surgery. In cases where I think radiation may be helpful I leave small metallic clips to guide the radiation oncologist to where the melanoma was located during the initial operation. This helps to maximize the dose of radiation to the sites that need treatment the most. The timing of radiation in relation to other adjuvant therapy must also be considered carefully.

Follow-Up Care for Stage IV Melanoma

In Stage IV melanoma, it is essential that regular scans are obtained to determine how effective treatment is for each patient. If that treatment is working it should be continued until the maximum benefit is reached—either complete disappearance of all melanoma in the best case, or a partial regression or shrinkage of melanoma, or stabilization with no change. If the treatment is not effective, most melanomas will grow and can double in size in as little as two months. Scans of the sites involved with melanoma should be obtained at least every two to three months. It is equally important to assess areas of the body that may be normal at the start of treatment to make sure that there is no evidence of new melanoma. Once the melanoma spreads to one site it can spread to any other site. For example, if the melanoma spreads to the lungs, it is important to make sure that the liver and brain are unaffected. An effective treatment should not only shrink melanoma but also prevent new melanoma from growing in other body organs.

The recommendations for following Stage IV patients are similar to those for Stage III patients. (See Table 10-4.) The frequency of scans may need to be adjusted for each patient, depending on how fast the melanoma is growing. This frequency is typically every two or three months. Those lucky patients who have a complete response to treatment should still follow the recommendations in Table 10-4.

There is less need for PET scans in Stage IV melanoma, although in selected cases it may be useful. When metastatic disease is detected by PET scan the area can be followed by repeated PET scans instead of CT scans. In addition, I routinely use PET scan in those patients whose melanoma shrinks to only one or two lesions by CT scan. I recommend surgical removal only when the PET scan shows no other melanoma. Furthermore, the PET scan can give us some clues as to how active the few remaining melanomas cells are. This may be important information, since treatments such as IL-2 may only destroy melanoma slowly and the CT scan may not return to normal for some time.

Although Stage IV melanoma patients should not forget about the skin and avoiding sun exposure, this is much less important than treating and following the metastatic disease. If the melanoma responds to treatment, attention is turned toward our usual recommendations for avoiding the sun and performing careful skin examinations.

Table 10-4. Follow-up recommendations for Stage IV melanoma patients

Recommendation	How Often?
Avoid sun exposure; use sunscreen	Daily if treatment is successful
Self skin examination	Once a month if treatment is successful
CT scan chest, abdomen, and pelvis	Every 2–3 months for 2 years, then every 6 months for 3 years, then as needed
Liver enzymes, LDH blood test	Every 3 months until disease resolves, then every 6 months for 5 years
Brain MRI	Every 3–6 months for 2 years, then once a year for 3 years, then as needed
Professional skin screening	Twice a year if treatment is successful
PET scan	As needed to evaluate other disease
Seek medical help for new lump or symptoms	As needed

Columbia Melanoma Center Case Studies

Larry had a Stage II melanoma on his right cheek removed by wide lo-cal excision when he was thirty-seven. He did not seek follow-up treat-ment. Two years later he happened to have a chest X-ray after getting into a minor traffic accident. The chest X-ray revealed a small lesion in his right lung. A chest CT scan showed two nodules in the right lung and one in the left lung. A biopsy of the left lung lesion confirmed melanoma and he came to the Melanoma Center for treatment.

I started him on IL-2 therapy and within a few months all the melanoma in Larry's lung had disappeared except for one small lesion that was half its original size. I ordered a PET scan to determine how active this melanoma was and to make sure there were no other areas of melanoma in the body. The PET scan showed activity in the small right lung melanoma, but no other melanoma elsewhere. I therefore recommended that Larry have surgery to remove the lung melanoma. A thoracoscopic procedure in which small incisions are made in the side of the chest removed the melanoma. He recovered well with no complications.

Larry returned to the center after his operation for follow-up care. I advised him to have a CT scan of the chest, abdomen, and pelvis every three months for two years. In addition, he will have an MRI of the brain every six months. A blood test for liver enzymes and LDH will also be done every six months. I have been following Larry for two years now and there has been no evidence of recurrent melanoma. We will now do CT scans every six months and he will have twice yearly skin screenings. He also performs monthly skin examinations and avoids sun exposure.

Larry is a highly successful example of how individualized planning can be effective for patients with Stage IV melanoma. If he had been followed after his first melanoma of the cheek, it might have been possible to detect the melanoma in the lung much earlier when surgery alone may have been effective. He is now aware of the importance of follow-up care and never misses an appointment.

Ask Your Doctor

If you have been treated for any stage of melanoma, ask the following questions:

1. *What is the plan for my follow-up care?* Every melanoma patient should have a clear plan for follow-up care after completing treatment for their melanoma. Ask your doctor for your plan. It should be based on the stage of your melanoma, your medical condition, and the ability to obtain appropriate tests at your hospital or clinic.

2. *What imaging tests do I need?* Except for Stage I melanoma where no

specific imaging tests are needed, all patients should have regular imaging for at least five years after treatment. This may be a simple chest X-ray once a year for low risk Stage II melanoma patients or CT scans every two months for metastatic patients. Your doctor may feel that PET scan is better for your particular melanoma. This should be clarified and incorporated into the overall follow-up plan. Ask your doctor what his or her reasoning is for using one test over the other one. You should be able to understand the rationale and participate in developing the plan.

3. *What blood tests do I need?* At a minimum most melanoma patients should have liver enzymes and LDH levels tested. Remember, any elevation of enzymes should prompt full-body CT scans to look for recurrent melanoma. Your doctor should explain if other blood tests will be done and you should be clear about how often these will be obtained.

4. *Who will review my test results?* As part of the follow-up plan you should decide which doctor will review your results and contact you with the outcome of all studies. Your choice may depend on your preference and how comfortable your primary care physician is with melanoma. Ask about this so there are no misunderstandings.

5. *Who will perform skin examinations?* Since the diagnosis of melanoma requires lifelong skin examination you should be referred to a specialist who knows how to do such examinations. Clarify who will be in charge of these examinations so that one professional, whether a dermatologist or a melanoma expert, can get to know you, your skin, and your moles.

CHAPTER ELEVEN

How to Control Melanoma Pain

A LTHOUGH PAIN IS one of the most dreaded symptoms of melanoma, it does not always occur. Still, concerns about pain merit special attention as it can complicate treatment and, most important, can usually be alleviated. Once the source of pain is diagnosed, appropriate treatment can be instituted as soon as possible. There is never a good reason to suffer from pain for any prolonged period of time.

What Is Pain?

Pain is a perception that something is wrong with the body, and it can be caused by many factors. Injury to the body can trigger painful sensations that are carried by nerve fibers to parts of the brain. The brain interprets these nerve impulses as pain. Painful stimuli can be significantly influenced by past experiences, mood, expectation, depression, cultural experiences, and genetics.

Several different types of pain exist. **Somatic pain** is directly related to signals received from nerves throughout the skin and muscles and is experienced most often as a sharp or aching sensation in a specific site on the body. Sometimes somatic pain feels like throbbing or pressure from outside the body. This is the type of pain you would feel if you hit your thumb with a hammer. In contrast, **visceral pain** comes from swelling of the internal organs, usually resulting from an obstruction. Visceral pain is crampy, diffuse, and difficult to pinpoint. Bad stomach flu or kidney stones cause visceral pain. A third type of pain is **neuropathic pain.** Neuropathic pain can be very severe but is localized along the distribution of a nerve. For example, sciatica occurs when the sciatic nerve is compressed, causing neuropathic pain down the back of the leg. The nerves that produce neuropathic pain can include a single nerve close to the skin, a collection of nerves closer to the spinal cord, or the spinal cord itself. Neuropathic pain usually results from melanoma putting pressure on a nerve or nerve bundle.

Pain can also be divided into acute and chronic pain. **Acute pain** develops suddenly in a previously normal person. Acute pain may be associated with high blood pressure, rapid pulse, and sweating. **Chronic pain** lasts for prolonged periods of time and does not change in quality or intensity. Chronic pain sufferers don't have the physical changes of acute pain as the body adjusts to having pain. However, depression, anxiety, insomnia, and anorexia may occur if chronic pain is left untreated.

A common feature of cancer-related pain is **breakthrough pain,** a sudden escalation from chronic pain to acute pain. Breakthrough pain may be a complication of treatment or may happen because of daily activities that cause further pressure or injury to damaged areas, such as bearing weight on a diseased bone, having a bowel movement, or coughing. Pain that occurs spontaneously with a short stabbing or lightning-like quality is characteristic of breakthrough pain. Breakthrough pain may also occur if the pain medications wear off before the next dose is due. Increasing the dose of medication or taking medication more frequently usually eliminates such breakthrough pain.

There are many sources of pain if you have melanoma. Some of the more common cancer pain syndromes are described in Table 11-1. Although the list is long, an oncologist with experience in diagnosing and treating cancer pain can control pain.

Table 11-1. Common cancer pain syndromes

Pain Syndrome	Type of Pain	Symptoms	Cause
Pathologic fracture	Somatic	Sudden, sharp, unrelenting pain over an area of bone	Melanoma in bone
Bowel obstruction	Visceral	Intermittent abdominal cramps; may also have constipation, nausea, and vomiting	Melanoma blocking the bowels
Bile duct obstruction	Visceral	Intermittent pain in the right upper part of the abdomen or right flank; jaundice (yellowing of skin)	Melanoma blocking the bile duct
Renal outflow obstruction	Visceral	Intermittent pain in lower abdomen or flank, blood in urine; rarely problems with kidney function	Melanoma blocking the ureters (tubes from kidneys to bladder) or bladder
Infection	Non-specific	Pneumonia is most common, with pain on breathing, cough, fever, chills	Melanoma blocking respiratory tract
Post-operative pain	Somatic	Pain or aching sensation in area of surgical incision; sometimes numbness and may involve the arms or legs	Damage of a peripheral nerve in the area of the surgical scar
Peripheral neuropathy	Neuropathic	Painful numbness or tingling, most commonly involving the hands and feet	Complication of chemotherapy (such as cisplatin)
Peripheral nerve damage	Neuropathic	Constant burning pain over the area of skin served by a single nerve	Melanoma invading a peripheral nerve

Pain Syndrome	Type of Pain	Symptoms	Cause
Spinal cord syndrome	Neuropathic	Pain, numbness, or weakness in the arms or legs, loss of bowel and bladder control	Melanoma placing pressure on the spinal cord or nerves extending out from the spinal cord
Plexopathy	Neuropathic	Severe unrelenting pain in the head, neck, arms, abdomen, pelvis, or legs	Melanoma invading the area where nerves come together before going to the spinal cord ("plexus")

What Causes Pain If You Have Melanoma?

People with advanced melanoma may experience pain from somatic, visceral, or neuropathic sources. The most common cause of melanoma pain is metastasis involving the bone; other causes are listed in Table 11-1. A growing body of research suggests that pain due to cancer is not essentially different than pain from other causes, though most patients perceive pain due to cancer as much worse.

Pain and the stage of disease are related. In early stages, pain is unusual and most often associated with treatment, such as typical postoperative incision pain. Stage IV patients are the most likely to experience cancer-related pain. Despite the relationship of the stage of melanoma to the intensity of the pain, there is no correlation with the amount of melanoma and the likelihood of pain. The location of the melanoma and its disruption of normal structures may be the culprit for most melanoma-related pain.

While most pain is due to the melanoma, it is also possible that pain may be unrelated. Some people will develop pain as a result of treatment, including surgery, chemotherapy, immunotherapy, and radiation therapy, which can damage normal tissue and cause pain. Likewise, some patients may develop pain from other causes, such as arthritis. The distinction between the causes is important since the treatment may differ depending on the source of the pain.

Recurrence or growth of the melanoma should be suspected whenever a worsening or change in existing pain occurs. This may require new imaging or other interventions. If the worst fears are confirmed, they may indicate a change in treatment plan. It is important always to inform your doctor of new pain or changes in the quality or intensity of previous pain.

How Can Pain Be Treated?

The good news is that most melanoma-related pain can be effectively controlled or treated. The first step is to diagnose the source of the pain and determine its intensity. The intensity of pain can be measured in a variety of ways. A common method is to ask patients to describe the pain on a scale of 1–10, so that the intensity of treatment can be adjusted to match the intensity of the pain. A numerical description is also helpful for determining how well a particular treatment is working. The treatment selected is individualized for each patient and depends on the cause of the pain, the intensity of the pain, the ability of patients to tolerate certain medications, and the proper treatment of related conditions, such as depression.

If you have pain you should see your doctor, who may be able to tell a lot about the source of the pain by talking to you and doing a physical examination. Imaging studies help determine whether melanoma is present at a painful site. Simple X-rays often help detect melanoma in the bone as a source of pain. You should receive some sort of medication before the X-rays so that you are comfortable during the procedure. For most visceral pain, a CT scan of the chest, abdomen, and pelvis is necessary to identify melanoma in these internal organs as well as finding other potential problems. An MRI of the brain and/or spinal cord may be helpful for neuropathic pain. In addition, electrophysiology studies can determine if there is damage to a specific nerve.

The mainstay of pain control for melanoma is with medications. Minor pain may be easily controlled with a non-narcotic medication, such as a non-steroidal anti-inflammatory agent or Tylenol. If this method is ineffective, **opioid-based narcotics** are the treatment of choice. Although my patients often hear the word "narcotics" and become anxious about addiction, they need not worry if only using these drugs briefly to control cancer pain. Studies document that as many as 90 percent of cancer patients experience the relief of symptoms with opioid-based medications. For mild to moderate symptoms a weak opioid may be selected, but for intense pain a strong opioid is the treatment of choice.

The single best drug is **morphine.** For patients in significant pain I start morphine as soon as possible, rather than letting the pain grow out of control while trying less effective narcotic agents. Morphine can be given by mouth for immediate action or as a sustained release tablet. The sustained release form is typically given every twelve hours and will provide long-lasting relief. However, the effects may wear off before the full twelve hours is over, especially when first starting the medication. If breakthrough pain occurs when starting on sustained relief morphine, immediate acting tablets or liquid provide complete pain relief. In severe pain syndromes, morphine can be given intravenously for even more rapid effects. The side effects of morphine include sleepiness, constipation, nausea, itchiness, and, rarely, respiratory distress. It may be best to start at a lower dose and slowly increase the dose until the pain is controlled. This approach is associated with few serious side effects. The constipation can be prevented by the early use of stool softeners, such as Colace, and fiber supplements, such as Metamucil, Senna, or other laxatives.

For patients who experience breakthrough pain on morphine or for those who may not be able to tolerate morphine, we can try other narcotics such as oxycodone, fentanyl, and methadone. Fentanyl is especially useful because it comes as a skin patch. The patch, which needs to be replaced every three days, provides similar pain control as morphine and does not require frequent doses of medication. The patch generally comes in twenty-five-microgram doses and should be adjusted up to an adequate dose. The starting dose depends on how severe the pain is at the time and your response to the patch. If there is no initial response, the dose of the patch can be increased or additional oral medication can be given. The patch often takes several days to achieve its full effect, so you may need some oral medications for support in the interim. Fentanyl is also available as a lollipop, so that the drug is absorbed under the tongue.

Oxycodone is an oral tablet that provides good pain control. It is not as potent as morphine for most melanoma-related pain but is useful for breakthrough or minor pain. The efficacy of oxycodone may be affected by abnormalities of kidney and liver function so should be used carefully in patients with kidney or liver disease. Methadone is a relatively safe alternative to morphine and is not affected by kidney function. If any of these medications cause toxicity, it is possible to switch to a different one.

The use of narcotics requires close supervision by a physician familiar with cancer patients. Inform your doctor of how you responded to each pain intervention and any new pain or other symptoms. It is normal to take several days or even weeks to adjust medications for optimal pain relief.

What if the narcotics are not enough? You have several options. A non-steroidal anti-inflammatory agent can help alleviate pain used together with morphine, fentanyl, and other narcotic agents. *Naproxen* is given only twice a day and is fairly inexpensive. *Tylenol* is also an excellent choice, and an extra-strength Tylenol every four to six hours can significantly improve pain control with morphine or other narcotics. Additional medications may be used in specific cases. Corticosteroids can control pain and may also help limit nausea, vomiting, and stimulate appetite. Corticosteroids should *not* be given to melanoma patients who have received or are contemplating immunotherapy because cortico-steroids can reverse the effects of immunotherapy. **Bisphosphonates** can prevent the breakdown of bone. These medications were originally used to lower calcium levels and prevent osteoporosis, but have worked well for painful bone metastases. **Calcitonin,** a hormone produced by the thyroid gland, lowers calcium levels. Calcitonin may also decrease bone pain and has been used in cases resistant to other treatments.

Surgery may provide immediate pain relief and is most helpful for solitary melanoma lesions in or just below the skin, which can be easily removed. Surgery to remove an obstructing melanoma may relieve pain quickly when the melanoma is encroaching on the bowels, bile duct, or urinary tubes. This kind of surgery, called palliative surgery, will only relieve symptoms and not address the overall disease process. Even when the surgery is successful there is a high likelihood that the melanoma will return to the same site so relief is often temporary. Therefore, palliative surgery for pain control should be reserved only for those situations in which the pain is unbearable and no other options have worked.

Radiation therapy can be remarkably effective for painful melanoma lesions, especially in the bone. A single high-dose treatment often re-sults in dramatic relief from pain, although it does not necessarily kill the melanoma completely. We think the radiation alters the inflammatory factors being released by the melanoma enough to lessen or entirely pre-vent the pain. Radiation therapy should be used early, especially when there are only a few painful areas, since this will easily and rapidly re-verse pain.

While most somatic and visceral pain responds well to the treatments I've discussed, neuropathic pain can be more difficult to treat. If it does not respond to morphine and other narcotics, additional approaches may be considered. A **lidocaine patch** releases lidocaine, a local anes-thetic, into the skin. It neutralizes the activity of nearby nerves and may offer immediate relief if pain is due to a single peripheral nerve close to the skin. **Tricyclic anti-depressants** may also alleviate neuropathic pain and are worth trying. Anti-seizure medications, such as **valproic acid,** may be beneficial in selected cases. If all else fails, a **nerve block** may be useful. In a nerve block, alcohol is injected at the site of the nerve plexus. A nerve block's success depends on the accuracy of the diagnosis and the skill of the physician performing the injection.

Growing evidence indicates alternative medicine approaches work for pain control, especially as adjuncts and to help with breakthrough pain. I advocate all patients consider alternative approaches, but not in place of more proven medications. The Melanoma Center has an alternative medicine office that you can consult for information on hypnosis, biofeedback, image-guided relaxation, aromatherapy, acupuncture, and other techniques (see also Chapter 14).

Many large medical centers have special pain management teams to help patients with chronic pain. These teams may be able to recommend new options if you continue to experience pain despite the treatments mentioned above.

Table 11-2. General treatment options for melanoma-related pain

Treatment	Comments
Radiation therapy	Single fraction doses are very effective for bone and soft tissue metastases
Narcotics	Most effective agents for typical pain; morphine and fentanyl patch
Non-steroidal anti-inflammatory agents	For selected breakthrough pain; naproxen most widely used agent
Tylenol	For breakthrough pain
Lidocaine patch	For neuropathic pain
Anti-depressants	For treating underlying depression, which helps with pain control and for neuropathic pain

Treatment	Comments
Anti-seizure medications	For neuropathic pain
Nerve blocks	For some types of neuropathic pain
Surgery	May be useful in selected cases to remove a painful melanoma lesion
Alternative methods	Hypnosis, biofeedback, aromatherapy, and image-guided relaxation techniques are helpful in many patients
Adjuvant medications	Corticosteroids; bisphosphonates and calcitonin may reduce bone pain

Other Concerns for Advanced Melanoma Patients

Appetite Loss

A major problem for advanced melanoma patients is their loss of appetite and accompanying rapid weight loss. Appetite stimulants such as Megace, Ritalin, or corticosteroids can increase your desire for food. Several small meals a day may be more effective than forcing someone to eat three large meals. I encourage patients to eat things they enjoy, which is the best way of nourishing them. High-calorie nutritional products such as Ensure can supplement the diet as well.

Depression

Depression and anxiety are normal responses to finding out that you have cancer. You may also get frustrated when one particular treatment doesn't work. While this is a normal reaction, severe depression can interfere with the doctor's ability to evaluate and treat the patient. It also affects many body functions, including appetite, sleep patterns, and mood. There is no shame in admitting that you may be depressed or feeling hopeless. These feelings can often be easily reversed with a short course of anti-depressants. Talk to your doctor about depression early, even if you are not feeling depressed all the time.

Fatigue

You may feel tired during or after treatment. While it is possible that melanoma alone may induce extreme fatigue, many times it is related to other factors. Anemia, for example, may be caused by the melanoma, chemotherapy, or result from something else. Anemia can be detected by a simple blood test that measures the number of red blood cells and is reported routinely as part of the complete blood count. Anemia can be corrected by iron supplementation in mild cases. If it's more extensive, usually when the anemia is related to chemotherapy, Procrit can be used. Procrit induces more red blood cell formation in the bone marrow and can reverse anemia. The medication is given as a small injection just under the skin once a week until the anemia improves. In severe cases of anemia, a blood transfusion provides immediate relief. Fatigue is a complication of almost all treatments used for melanoma, so some degree of tiredness may be expected after therapy. This should clear in a few weeks in most cases. Fatigue may also be a side effect of narcotic medications and sometimes a reduced dose of medicine will improve the fatigue. If you experience fatigue, notify your doctor so that the source can be identified. Even when a specific cause cannot be identified, medications such as Ritalin and corticosteroids may alleviate fatigue and encourage well-being.

Sleep

Patients with melanoma often experience changes in their sleep habits. Insomnia or increasing sleepiness may be a symptom of underlying depression or anxiety and will greatly diminish once those are treated. Sleep disturbances may be related to therapy, as happens frequently with high-dose IL-2. Sleep disturbances are also quite common in end-stage melanoma and can be a concern for many patients. Discuss sleep changes with your doctor to determine the cause. Treating the cause will improve sleep patterns, or a short course of medication may help.

End-Stage Considerations

As much as I want to help patients fight advanced melanoma for as long as possible, I try to be aware of when it's time to stop. When I know we've run out of options, then my role shifts to making patients as comfortable as possible. In addition to aggressive pain control, addressing depression, sleep, and fatigue in the ways I've already discussed can help ease a patient's end of life.

Another subject that may come up with end-stage melanoma patients is their inability to make decisions. This may happen because of confusion from melanoma in the brain or complications of treatment. Designating a health care proxy who is able to make informed decisions on your behalf can give you some peace of mind. Many states now require this of all patients in a hospital, but even if your state doesn't, it is a good idea when you have Stage IV melanoma. A health proxy should be a person who knows you well and understands your desires and wishes. Your health care proxy should know if you would prefer home hospice care to hospital care, for example. A hospice can arrange support for patients and their families when a patient wishes to die at home. Your doctor can work with the hospice to make sure that you are adequately medicated to prevent pain.

Although I am optimistic about treating melanoma, in cases where a cure is unlikely, I want you to remember that your doctor can improve your quality of life. The measures that we can employ after stopping treatment are just as important for your well-being. Understanding the issues and knowing how to make patients more comfortable is also crucial for family members dealing with this sad situation.

Columbia Melanoma Center Case Studies

Frank was a twenty-eight-year-old man who arrived at the Center with metastatic melanoma in the lungs, liver, bone, and multiple soft tissue sites. He had no response to the first treatment I tried, high-dose IL-2. I then tried chemotherapy, again with no luck. An experimental vaccine in a clinical trial did no good either. Frank then developed severe pain in one of his melanoma lesions. Initially treated with morphine, the pain continued to worsen. He also complained of feeling tired and had severe constipation. I removed the melanoma lesion surgically, and his pain quickly disappeared. Stopping the morphine led to improvement in his constipation and fatigue. He was actually able to go back to work for several weeks.

Then he complained of lower back pain, and a CT scan showed new melanoma lesions in the lower vertebrae. After radiation therapy, the pain resolved as well. Over the next two months Frank became increasingly tired and lost his appetite. Although anti-depressant drugs, appetite stimulating medications, and nutritional supplements helped him feel better, his melanoma continued to grow. Frank and his wife came to the Center to discuss his options. Together, we decided that he would be most comfortable at home. I prescribed him a fentanyl patch and oral medications for breakthrough pain. A local hospice representative helped the family set up a special bed to relieve the pressure on Frank's lower back.

Frank passed away at home and his wife came back to let us know that his last few weeks were comfortable and peaceful.

Ask Your Doctor

If you are experiencing pain, ask the following questions:

1. *What is causing the pain?* Before developing any treatment plan, it is important to know the cause of the pain. After examining you, your doctor should have some ideas about the cause, and sometimes additional X-rays or scans are needed to confirm the source of pain.

2. *What is the plan for pain control?* If the pain is due to melanoma, you have many options for pain control, depending on the pain's location, type, and intensity. Make sure you understand how your medications are used, the dosage, and the potential side effects. Consult with your doctor to develop a back-up plan for pain control, and also ask about breakthrough pain and its treatment.

3. *What if the plan is not successful?* Your doctor will probably have a back-up plan, should the initial regimen prove unsuccessful. Many patients are relieved to know that there are other options. Give the current regimen every chance to work first, but also be aware of Plan B.

4. *Should we stop active treatment?* This is perhaps the most difficult choice of all. When making this decision, take into account the realistic likelihood of successful treatment, side effects of treatment, quality of life without treatment, and the range of palliative measures available. This decision should involve your wishes, as well as your family's, and be made in consultation with your doctor. Know what alternatives are available if you choose to stop active treatment.

5. *What are some resources for end of life care?* Most centers have some source of support for patients and their families when they decide to stop treatment. A hospice can be reached at 800-854-3402, or through the Hospice Foundation of America Web site at www.hospicefoundation.org, if your hospital does not have a local office. Many centers have social workers, psychologists, or nurse specialists who can provide resources for patients electing home care.

PART FOUR

Melanoma Research

CHAPTER TWELVE

New Cytokine Therapy Research

MELANOMA TREATMENT IS far from perfect, especially for patients with Stage III and IV disease. While certain treatments do help patients, even curing some with Stage IV melanoma, the number of patients who stay well is much too low. But exciting research is helping to find better treatments for this disease. Two major breakthroughs have helped move us closer to that goal within the last few years.

First is the sequencing of the human genome, an amazing accomplishment that means scientists now have the exact DNA coding sequence for all human genes. An understanding of the genetic make-up of humans is leading to new insights into why melanoma cells behave the way they do. This research has already led to new drugs for correcting abnormalities in melanoma cells. New cytokines, similar to interferon and interleukin-2, have been identified. Discovering new immune system genes has led to tremendous excitement about developing vaccines for treatment, or possibly even prevention, of melanoma. The identification of abnormal genes or gene function in melanoma cells is also leading to new drugs that correct these abnormalities.

The second major breakthrough is high throughput screening, a method for testing new genes and drugs in large batches allowing very rapid retrieval of results. Being able to screen or analyze new drugs so quickly allows us to pick a winner much more easily and accurately than ever before. All such new drugs must first be tested, and that's where

clinical trials come in. While clinical trials can never guarantee an outcome, they are an option for many patients for whom other treatments
have failed.

Cytokine Research

The cytokines are molecules produced by the immune system that
help to turn immune responses on and off. These molecules have been
extensively studied in the laboratory and synthetic, or man-made, copies
are available for many cytokines. The cytokines have powerful effects
in patients and have proven to be valuable in the treatment of cancer. In fact, two cytokines, interferon-alpha and interleukin-2, have been
approved for the treatment of melanoma.

Research in my field today is focusing on how to optimize inter-
leukin-2 (IL-2) for melanoma therapy, reduce its side effects, and identify other cytokines that may be beneficial for melanoma treatment. In
this chapter I review the current research related to new cytokines and
some of the approaches under investigation for improving the existing
cytokines. While not every cytokine will ultimately prove useful for
melanoma treatment, new drugs and new strategies may emerge from
this research.

Research to Improve Interferon-alpha

Interferon-alpha is a cytokine, a substance produced by cells of the
immune system that helps to activate the immune response. Interferon
was named because of its ability to "interfere" with the replication of
viruses. Interferon-alpha as a treatment is a man-made compound (or
synthetic drug) that is an exact copy of naturally occurring interferon.
Interferon has many actions that may help to fight melanoma and other
cancer cells. Interferon causes direct death to cancer cells and also activates the immune response against cancers. At low doses, interferon-
alpha also shuts down blood vessel growth that cancers need for survival.

All of these effects may contribute to the beneficial clinical effects from interferon in patients with melanoma.

Interferon-alpha has been approved for high-risk melanoma patients since late 1995 but remains a difficult treatment regimen due to the high incidence of severe side effects and the need to be on therapy for up to one year. In an effort to limit the side effects associated with long-term interferon treatment investigators are evaluating a number of new strategies, which include delivering interferon in slow-release formulations. A process called **pegylation** results in a slow sustained release of the drug after injection and, hence, lower levels of circulating interferon. This appears to decrease the risk of side effects, although further studies are needed to determine if this kind of formulation also has clinical activity against melanoma.

There is also on-going research to try lower doses of interferon and shorter time schedules of interferon therapy. However, we must wait for these studies to be completed before changing the currently recommended dose and schedule of interferon-alpha.

Other researchers are attempting to determine exactly how interferon-alpha fights melanoma. This research is especially important as it may provide new insights into how to make interferon therapy better and less toxic. Similarly, this area of research may be able to suggest new combinations that will be particularly effective for melanoma and perhaps other cancers as well.

Research to Improve Interleukin-2 (IL-2)

Interleukin-2 is a naturally occurring molecule made by T cells that helps to promote T-cell survival and activation. Large amounts of IL-2 are made during infections with a virus, and it helps to provide new T cells and improve their killing activity. This may be beneficial not just for infections, but also for cancer and for increasing the number of CD4+ T cells in patients with HIV infection. A man-made, or synthetic, form of IL-2 is also available for treatment.

High dose IL-2 remains the best treatment option for those patients with metastatic melanoma who can tolerate the treatment. Since the side effects of high-dose IL-2 are a major problem, several approaches have been evaluated in an attempt to reduce the incidence of such side effects. Despite many trials using lower doses of IL-2, the clinical effects have not been comparable to those observed with the higher doses. Therefore, lowering the dose is not usually acceptable.

Other strategies have been explored for trying to decrease the side effects while allowing administration of the standard high doses of IL-2. To date there has been little progress in this area, although scientists continue to pursue new drugs that help control the blood pressure and other side effects commonly seen with IL-2 administration.

An interesting strategy for improving the clinical effects of IL-2 has been to combine IL-2 with other treatments or drugs with demonstrated activity against melanoma. In fact, IL-2 has been tested in combination with interferon-alpha and with many different chemotherapy regimens. Unfortunately, most of these clinical trials have not shown any additional benefit when compared with high-dose IL-2 alone.

As we will see in Chapter 13, vaccines have become very promising and these work by stimulating the immune system to attack melanoma, in a manner similar to IL-2. Preliminary experiments in animals have shown that IL-2 can significantly improve the response against cancer, such as melanoma, when given in combination with a vaccine. This concept is being tested in clinical trials for patients with melanoma. The ability to provide IL-2 in a local manner at the site of vaccination also appears to provide the maximum benefit of the combination while limiting the side effects of IL-2. It will be exciting to see the results of these studies in patients.

Granulocyte-Macrophage Colony Stimulating Factor (GM-CSF)

Granulocyte-macrophage colony stimulating factor, or GM-CSF, is a member of the colony stimulating factor family. These are naturally occurring cytokines that help to induce the growth of specific types of blood cells. Thus, GM-CSF acts to turn early bone marrow cells into white blood cells, including granulocytes, macrophages, and eosinophils, all different types of blood cells. In addition, GM-CSF is a powerful stimulus for dendritic cells, which are important cells for starting an immune response.

GM-CSF has been made in synthetic form and was initially used as a way to increase the number of white blood cells in patients who received chemotherapy or underwent a bone marrow transplant. More recently, GM-CSF has been used to help vaccines since the GM-CSF attracts dendritic cells to sites of vaccination and helps to start the immune response. In general, GM-CSF is given as a subcutaneous injection in the skin, similar to an insulin injection.

In a study conducted several years ago, patients with melanoma were treated with GM-CSF alone without any other therapy. The patients in this study had both Stage III and Stage IV melanoma. Overall the patients treated with GM-CSF lived longer than a group of patients who did not have GM-CSF, although the patients were not studied together. New clinical trials are being conducted to see if GM-CSF really has activity against melanoma alone or when given with a vaccine. These studies will be important to monitor to get a better idea of just how effective GM-CSF may be in melanoma.

The side effects of GM-CSF are well known and relatively minor, especially when compared to those side effects observed with interferon-alpha or interleukin-2. The common side effects are listed in Table 12-1. Most patients tolerate treatment with GM-CSF very well.

COMMON SIDE EFFECTS OF GM-CSF

- Headache
- Fever
- Chills
- Weakness
- Muscle Pain
- Bone Pain
- Rash

Interleukin-12

Interleukin-12 (IL-12) is a cytokine that is very similar to IL-2 and acts on both T cells and natural killer, or NK, cells. IL-12 is produced by dendritic cells and T cells. It acts as a growth factor for the T and NK cells, resulting in their activation and function as killer cells against both viruses and cancer. IL-12 also causes the cells to produce interferon-gamma, which is another cytokine that appears to be important for fighting cancer. In some studies IL-12 appears to be more powerful than IL-2 in activating T cells, and this led to its experimental use as a cytokine for treating cancer. A large number of animal models supported the strong anti-cancer properties of IL-12, leading to a great deal of interest in using IL-12 in patients.

The first clinical trials have been completed, and they further suggest that IL-12 may have some activity in treating cancer. These early studies included patients with melanoma. The responses observed thus far appear to be similar or slightly lower than those seen with high doses of IL-2. There are significant side effects associated with IL-12 administration, although they appear to be manageable, especially at lower doses. IL-12 has been given by both intravenous and subcutaneous injections; further research is needed to see just how effective IL-12 will be for melanoma.

There is also interest in combining IL-12 with other treatments, including IL-2. Early clinical studies have shown that this combination is relatively safe, and evidence of activity against melanoma has been reported. The ultimate role of IL-12 and other cytokines depends on continued clinical trials and investigation to determine the level of activity against melanoma and to optimize the proper dose and schedule of administration.

Interleukin-15

Interleukin-15 (IL-15) is a new cytokine that has activity on T cells similar to IL-2. An interesting point about IL-15 is that it is found in several different types of tissue throughout the body. IL-15 stimulates the growth of T cells, B cells, and NK cells. There is some research showing that IL-15 can even improve the survival of cancer specific T cells. IL-15 has been reported to be important for the survival of memory T cells, those T cells that remain in the body and are ready to deal with infections when the body is re-exposed after an initial infection. The fact that IL-15 is found in so many different tissues has suggested that it may function to keep T cells alive and active as they travel the body in search of infectious viruses or cancer cells. Because of this important activity and the similarities with IL-2, there is great hope for IL-15 as a clinical agent. Clinical trials need to be conducted to see just how effective IL-15 will be in treating patients with melanoma.

Interleukin-18

Interleukin-18 (IL-18) is another cytokine with many functions. IL-18 is similar to IL-12 and helps to stimulate T cells. In the body, IL-18 comes from activated monocytes in the blood and macrophages in the tissues of the body. Like IL-12, IL-18 acts on T cells and produces a number of other cytokines, including interferon-gamma, IL-2, and GM-CSF, all thought to have activity against cancer. IL-18 also enhanced the killing activity of T cells and NK cells. Many scientists believe that IL-18 plays a role in regulating the T-cell responses against viruses and cancers. Early studies in mice have shown activity against a wide variety of cancers, including melanoma. Clinical studies must be conducted to fully study the effects of IL-18 in patients with melanoma.

Table 12-1. Cytokines approved or being developed for melanoma treatment

Cytokine	Animal Models	Clinical Trials	Comment
Interferon-alpha	Yes	Yes	FDA approved for Stage III melanoma
Interleukin-2	Yes	Yes	FDA approved for Stage IV melanoma and kidney cancer
Granulocyte-macrophage colony stimulating factor	Yes	In progress	
Interleukin-12	Yes	In progress	
Interleukin-15	Yes	No	Trials expected
Interleukin-18	Yes	In progress	
Interleukin-21	Yes	No	
Interleukin-23	Yes	No	

Interleukin-21

Recently, interleukin-21 (IL-21) was identified as a member of the IL-2 family. IL-21 is produced by activated T-cells and helps to induce antibody formation, T-cell, and NK cell responses. The overall effect is to help activate an immune response. An important difference from IL-2 is that IL-21 may keep the immune response going for many days and thus could be more potent than IL-2. In preliminary animal studies IL-21 reduces the growth of cancers and improves survival of mice with cancer.

Interleukin-23

A newly described cytokine, interleukin-23 (IL-23), is related to IL-12 and is released in infected or damaged body tissues. Exposure to IL-23 causes T cells to divide and secrete other cytokines. In animals, IL-23 can prevent the growth of melanoma but clinical trials in patients have not been done. Undoubtedly, other cytokines will be identified with potential for treatment of melanoma.

I HAVE DISCUSSED some of the more promising cytokine candidates, and it is likely that many others will be discovered over the next few years. If we continue to conduct basic and clinical investigations into the effects that these cytokines have on the immune system and against melanoma, our treatment options will greatly expand.

Columbia Melanoma Center Case Studies

Virginia is a fifty-one-year-old woman who noticed a pigmented lesion growing in size on her left foot. A biopsy revealed an intermediate thickness melanoma and she underwent a wide local resection without complications. A sentinel lymph node biopsy was positive for melanoma in a single lymph node and she had a lymph node dissection. After surgery she considered interferon-alpha therapy but was unable to tolerate the side effects after one week of treatment. She was referred to the Melanoma Center to consider other adjuvant therapy options. After discussing the options Virginia decided to become a candidate for a study of GM-CSF cytokine therapy. She received GM-CSF and has been doing well for the last two years.

Ask Your Doctor

If you are interested in cytokine therapy, ask the following questions:

1. *Are there any cytokine studies available for my type of melanoma?* If your melanoma has not responded to standard therapy or if you are unable to tolerate interferon-alpha or IL-2 treatment, there may be other clinical trials in which you can participate. If your doctor is not aware of any current studies, read Chapter 15 and find out where such studies are being conducted. You usually need to meet several eligibility requirements before you will be able to enter a clinical study and most participating sites can give you information on whether you may qualify.

2. *What is the current status of cytokine therapy for melanoma?* Research changes quickly and it is difficult even for the experts to keep up on the new developments. Ask your doctor about the latest news in cytokine research and see if it may be appropriate for your situation.

3. *What are the side effects of cytokine treatment?* One of the goals of clinical research is to determine what the side effects are for any new drug, and cytokines are no exception. Each cytokine has a unique profile of side effects. You should review these with your doctor, whether you are considering a "standard" cytokine, such as IL-2 or interferon, or an experimental cytokine still in development.

4. *Where can I get more information on cytokine treatments?* If your doctor is not sure about the latest developments, he or she may be able to direct you to another physician who may be more up to date with this field. Many large tertiary centers have physicians with an interest in cytokine therapy, and they may be able to speak with you and your doctor about new clinical studies and additional treatment options.

CHAPTER THIRTEEN

Vaccine Therapy Research

MELANOMA IS A unique cancer because under some circumstances the immune system seems able to destroy melanoma cells. In rare situations, the immune system may entirely eradicate the melanoma, a condition referred to as a spontaneous regression. Even short of a complete regression, we often observe under the microscope a large number of T cells within melanomas. This indicates that the immune system—and T cells, in particular—do try to eliminate melanoma. But how does this happen? What activates the T cells in the first place? Why is it not effective in every patient? How can we develop better treatments for melanoma? The answers to these questions are the basis for vaccine therapy research.

Considerable evidence points to the immune system recognizing melanoma through T cells. T cells are not able to directly "see" melanoma cells, but are able to see small fragments of proteins, or antigens, made in melanoma cells. T cells roam the body looking for these antigens. In general, T cells can distinguish between normal body proteins, which they leave alone, and abnormal proteins (or antigens) made by viruses, for example. When the T cells find these antigens, they destroy the cells that have them. In some cases this is good for you, as when the T cells fight off virus infections by killing those cells infected with the virus. In other cases it's detrimental, such as when T cells notice a transplanted organ as not being part of the body and attack it, a process called **rejection.**

In melanoma the situation is more complex. Antigens can be classified as strong or weak based on how similar the antigen is to the person's natural proteins. For example, a virus has very different proteins from humans and so most viral antigens are strong and elicit a strong immune response. In contrast, most melanoma proteins are normal body proteins and so it is difficult to get a T cell to react against the melanoma. However, some proteins are mutated, and this generates new antigens not found in normal melanocytes. This may be enough to get a T cell to respond. In other cases, proteins may be made at a higher than normal rate or at abnormal times during the cell's life, and this may also be enough to generate a T cell response.

Melanoma Antigens

The first melanoma antigen was discovered in 1991 by using T cells taken from melanoma patients and exposing them to various antigens until one antigen was noticed to cause activation of the T cells. This antigen was called melanoma associated gene 1, or MAGE-1. Many melanoma antigens have been identified since then. The discovery of these antigens suggested that T cells could be generated against melanoma cells, although the response may be weak. The antigens can be used in vaccines to increase the chances of activating an immune response.

Table 13-1. Common melanoma antigens

Antigen	Clinical Trials to Test Antigen as a Vaccine
MART-1 (also called Melan-A)	Yes
gp100	Yes
tyrosinase	Yes

Antigen	Clinical Trials to Test Antigen as a Vaccine
tyrosinase-related protein-1	Yes
tyrosinase-related protein-2	Yes
MAGE-1	Yes
MAGE-3	Yes
BAGE	No
NY-ESO-1	Yes
GAGE	No
CDK4	No
beta-catenin	No
CDC27	No
gangliosides	Yes

Vaccines

A vaccine is any agent that activates an immune response. The discovery of antigens allows the vaccine to target a single protein. This provides an ideal way to single out melanoma cells while leaving most normal cells alone, so the side effects are generally low. While no vaccines are approved in the United States for melanoma as of this writing, there is overwhelming evidence that they work in animals. One type of melanoma vaccine has been approved in Canada and Australia for patients. Thus, an intense effort to evaluate vaccines in clinical trials for patients with melanoma has begun. I will now discuss the many different types of vaccines that are being tested in clinical trials.

Peptide Vaccines

Since T cells recognize antigens as peptides, the most obvious vaccine is the peptide itself. Synthetic peptides are simple to make. A problem with peptide vaccines, however, is that the peptides bind to the human leukocyte antigen (HLA) molecules. Since every patient has a different set of HLA molecules, the peptides must be designed for the specific HLA molecule in a given patient. We all inherit one HLA molecule from our mother and one from our father. In some cases you may get the same HLA molecule from each parent. The class I HLA molecules are called A, B, and C. The class II HLA molecules are called D. Using a simple blood sample we can determine the HLA type for any patient and this information is frequently used before transplantation and when deciding on peptide vaccines for cancer patients. The most common HLA type in the United States is HLA A2 and so most peptide vaccines have been specific for patients with HLA A2 typing.

A large number of peptide vaccine clinical trials have been conducted using peptides derived from the antigens listed in Table 13-1. As mentioned, patients must have the appropriate HLA type so the peptide will bind to the patient's HLA molecule and trigger a T-cell response. Usually peptide vaccines are given with non-specific immune adjuvants and cytokines, such as GM-CSF or IL-2. Although peptide vaccines appear to be safe and can activate T cells, there is little proof to date that they are effective in treating patients with melanoma. Nonetheless, some patients have responded and more research is needed.

Heat Shock Protein Vaccines

Heat shock proteins are found in nearly all cells and bind peptides inside the cell to help transport them to the HLA molecules for "viewing" by T cells. Preliminary research has shown that vaccination with heat shock protein-peptide complexes results in an unusually strong immune response. This finding suggests a new strategy for tumor vaccines whereby specific antigens are not needed. The heat shock proteins can be removed directly from melanoma cells and then used for vaccination. These vaccines are in essence "designer vaccines" since they are specific for each individual patient. This vaccination appears to have a similar safety profile as peptide vaccines and is being evaluated in larger clinical trials. Early studies have demonstrated that heat shock vaccines can generate both T-cell and NK-cell responses with several clinical responses reported. A major disadvantage is the need for tumor tissue to extract the heat shock proteins, which may be a problem in patients with little tumor but at high risk for disease. Likewise, enough melanoma may not be available for vaccine production.

DNA Vaccines

In order to avoid the need for HLA restrictions, an entire gene can be administered by using a DNA vaccine. This vaccine contains the DNA of a specific melanoma antigen or other immune stimulatory genes. DNA vaccines tested in patients have a good safety profile but so far there has not been enough evidence that these vaccines are effective. The DNA vaccine research is focusing on combinations with other vaccines to improve the response rates.

Viral Vaccines

Viral vaccines for melanoma treatment offer several advantages. First, the virus itself, which may be natural or synthetic, can enhance immune responses. Second, the virus can be used to carry a number of genes, including melanoma antigens, that help to activate the immune response against melanoma. The vaccine tricks the immune system into thinking that the melanoma antigen is part of the virus and should be destroyed. T cells can be "taught" to target melanoma cells provided they still contain the antigen. Viral vaccines can be engineered to contain other helpful immune genes that help to activate T cells.

These vaccines can infect dendritic cells and activate T cells. They can also direct the immune response to the site of the melanoma by injecting the vaccine directly into a melanoma. Numerous studies are being conducted with a variety of different viruses. Viral vaccines appear to be safe but further research is needed to understand if they will be effective in treating melanoma or preventing melanoma recurrence.

Dendritic Cell Vaccines

The important role of dendritic cells in initiating immune responses has led to interest in using these cells as tumor vaccines. Dendritic cells can be collected from blood samples and grown in large numbers in the laboratory. When enough cells are created, they can be exposed to specific melanoma antigens or melanoma cells, again in the lab. After infusing the cells back into a patient, mature dendritic cells will be able to activate T cells. The dendritic cells have been mixed with specific peptides, DNA, viral vaccines, and even whole, killed melanoma cells. Several clinical trials tried dendritic-cell vaccines in the treatment of patients with metastatic melanoma. These studies have shown that dendritic-cell vaccination was well tolerated. Although the numbers of patients treated so far have been small, there is evidence of positive responses in some patients. New research is using small molecules, called chemokines, to activate dendritic cells in the body. This avoids the need for collecting and growing dendritic cells in the laboratory, which is often difficult, expensive, and unsuccessful. Another class of molecules, known as toll-like receptor agonists, bind to dendritic cells and activate them into mature antigen presenting cells. Several such agonists, such as Aldara cream, are now being tested as a method for directly activating dendritic cells in the body, near the site of growing melanomas.

Autologous and Allogeneic Whole-Cell Vaccines

Once melanoma cells are irradiated, they can no longer cause melanoma when given to a patient. Rather, they act as a vaccine triggering an immune response against the melanoma cells. In some cases the immune system will attack all melanoma cells. There are two general approaches to such whole-cell vaccines. Autologous vaccines are made from the patient's own melanoma and offer the advantage of using cells that contain the patient's own HLA-matched cells. However, the antigens present in these vaccines are weak. Another problem is that autologous cell vaccines require enough melanoma to make the vaccine. In allogeneic whole-cell vaccines, melanoma cells from another patient's melanoma or those grown in the laboratory are used for vaccine preparation. Surprisingly, these vaccines have been very efficient at generating an immune response and are in clinical testing. This vaccine likely works because a number of antigens are shared between the patient's melanoma and the allogeneic melanoma cells. Whole-cell vaccines are often given with a mixture of a non-specific immune adjuvant, such as bacillus Calmette-Guerin (BCG), or low doses of cyclophosphamide.

Another variation of the whole-cell vaccine is to design the melanoma cells used in the vaccine to produce a helper cytokine, such as the cytokines IL-2 or GM-CSF. There is evidence from animal studies that this results in a better immune response and more powerful treatment effects. This strategy is being tested in clinical trials for a variety of different cancers.

Adoptive Transfer Therapy

The ultimate goal of vaccine therapy is to develop a strong T-cell response capable of destroying all the melanoma in the body. What if the vaccines are not able to activate a large enough number of T cells? It appears that there is a struggle between the melanoma growing, trying to survive, and the immune system, where T cells are trying to contain the melanoma. If there are simply not enough T cells, the melanoma will win the battle. Much work in the vaccine area suggests that vaccines can stimulate some T cells but may not be able to generate the army of T cells needed to deal with most melanomas. One strategy is to activate T cells directly in the laboratory, grow a large number of these killer T cells, and then give them back to the patient. Amazingly, this seems to be quite effective and new strategies for getting the most active T cells are being evaluated.

Today, T cells can be generated in the laboratory by exposing T cells from a patient to a variety of vaccines. This can stimulate a T cell against specific melanoma antigens and once the cells are grown in large numbers they can be given back to patients.

New research in immunology suggests that the survival of adoptively transferred T cells may be better when the patient's natural T cells are already depleted. The reason for this is not entirely clear; it may be because such depletions get rid of suppressor T cells that block the effects of activated T cells. Another possibility is that the rules for T cell survival may be altered in settings where all the T cells are low. Whatever the reason, clinical trials are already under way to use chemotherapy for depleting T cells or other drugs to deplete the suppressor T cells and then give back T cells or vaccinate the patient with specific vaccines. While this is a promising development, the only way to determine how effective it will be is through clinical trials.

Controlling the Immune System: Beyond Vaccines

Our improved understanding of the immune system has led to new research in manipulating immune responses. Scientists now believe that T cells require several molecular signals to become activated. The primary signal is delivered by the antigen and targets a particular virus or tumor cell. However, other signals are less specific and come from a series of molecules referred to as co-stimulatory molecules because they are necessary for stimulation of T cells. The co-stimulatory molecules are naturally found on dendritic cells; this helps to explain why these cells are so effective at activating T cells. Co-stimulatory molecules can also be added to vaccines as a way to increase the likelihood of T-cell activation.

Researchers who focused on co-stimulatory molecules were in for another surprise. It appears that the T cell has developed different receptors for the co-stimulatory molecules. Some of the receptors provide signals for growth and production of cytokines, leading to an activated immune response. However, other receptors turn the T cell off. A complex interplay between signals determines how active a T cell will be when it sees its antigen.

The recognition of the on/off switches on T cells has resulted in several new and very powerful drugs that can either trigger or block individual T-cell receptors. Very strong immune responses can be generated or, conversely, overactive immune responses can be shut down. This research has been tested in animal systems and appears to work very well for treatment of cancer, transplantation, and autoimmunity (a condition where the immune system attacks the body). Continued research is necessary to fully understand this complex system and determine how to manipulate the system for treatment of disease.

New research in immunology has led to a variety of innovative vaccines and other strategies for the treatment of melanoma. While this area of research has been quite exciting, there are still questions that need to be answered. Many of these approaches need to be carefully evaluated in clinical trials. Although most vaccines have been safe thus far, as the vaccines become more powerful, new side effects, such as autoimmune disease, may be more likely. The development of vaccines for melanoma is a good example of how basic scientific research is leading to new treatments. The role of vaccines will depend on patients participating in clinical trials to help demonstrate the beneficial as well as adverse effects of each new agent.

Columbia Melanoma Center Case Studies

Nancy was sixty-two when she was referred to the Melanoma Center by her primary care doctor. She had been diagnosed with an intermediate thickness melanoma of her left foot when she was fifty-seven years old and was treated by local resection. However, in a routine physical examination her doctor noticed enlarged lymph nodes in her left groin, and a biopsy revealed melanoma. Nancy had a complete set of CT scans and melanoma was found in both lungs. She came to the Melanoma Center, and we considered several treatment options. Nancy was interested in a vaccine clinical trial, as she did not want chemotherapy and felt that she would not be able to tolerate high-dose IL-2. She was treated with a new poxvirus vaccine, which contains a co-stimulatory molecule. The vaccine was given directly into the melanoma in a left-groin lymph node since this was easily accessible. Nancy received three monthly vaccinations and was able to function normally after each office visit. After the third vaccination her lymph nodes began to regress and eventually disappeared. A repeat CT scan demonstrated that the melanoma in her lungs had also disappeared. Nancy noticed that while her melanoma had responded, she had developed a new area of whitish skin around her lower lip, vitiligo. Vitiligo is not a side effect of melanoma, but we think it is somehow related to the immunologic responses to melanoma treatment. Nancy has now been free of melanoma for three years. She uses extra make-up to cover the area of vitiligo around her lower lip.

Ask Your Doctor

If you are interested in vaccine therapy, ask the following questions:

1. *Am I a candidate for a vaccine study?* Many patients will be considered candidates for participation in a vaccine study. Typically, vaccine studies are considered only after some form of standard therapy fails, and many studies will require completion of standard therapy beforehand. In some cases, patients may not be able to

tolerate standard therapy or may refuse such treatment. In these cases vaccines may be an appealing possibility. Your doctor can help determine if you are eligible for such a trial.

2. *What is the vaccine?* As we have seen, there are numerous types of vaccines in testing today. Since there is no absolute proof that one vaccine is better than the other you can consider particular vaccines based on their own merits. Your doctor should be able to discuss the nature of the vaccine, how it is thought to work, and what the expected benefits and risks are from the vaccine.

3. *What is the plan if the vaccine fails?* Since not every patient will respond, it is acceptable to ask what additional treatments might be available in the event that the vaccine does not work.

4. *What is the plan if the vaccine works?* In some cases the vaccine will have a positive impact on the disease. This may be a complete response, but often there is a partial response or a stabilization of disease. You should discuss with your doctor what you will do in this situation. This can be a problem; some physicians would encourage other treatment to fight the disease and some would wait if the disease has stabilized. In this case, regular scans could detect when the disease begins to grow and allow you to save other treatment options for later.

5. *Should I be referred to a melanoma center?* If your doctor does not have vaccines and other experimental treatments, you may ask to be referred to a larger melanoma center where such treatment may be available.

CHAPTER FOURTEEN

Genetic and Targeted Therapy Research

ADVANCES IN MOLECULAR biology and immunology are leading to the development of an ever increasing number of new drugs and approaches for the treatment of melanoma. Although this field is always changing and new agents can be expected over the next decade, I will try to summarize a few of the important discoveries. As the medical research community gains experience with new drugs, further modifications and refinements will improve the quality of such agents. Furthermore, clinical testing often begins with studies of a single agent, which then expands to test various known drugs in new combinations. We can expect an increasing number of new drugs and combinations over the next several years. This chapter should be used as a guide to the basic principles underlying these new areas of research and a reference for the general approach, rather than as a statement on the effectiveness of any given agent.

Table 14-1 lists some of the new strategies being used for treatment, including specific drugs that have been tested in melanoma patients. In most cases the general approach has been tested in other types of cancer but may have some promise for melanoma.

Table 14-1. New treatment approaches for melanoma

General Strategy	How it works	Drugs Tested in Other Cancers	Drugs Tested in Melanoma
Immunotherapy	Monoclonal antibodies target specific molecules	Herceptin; Erbitux; Rituxan	Experimental
	Non-specific immune stimulants activate immune system	Thalomid; Revimid	Thalomid
Targeted therapy	Blocks signal transduction pathways in cancer cells	Gleevec	Raf kinase inhibitors
Gene therapy	Gene inserted into cancer cells stops growth or activates immune system	Experimental	Experimental
Anti-angiogenesis	Blocks new blood vessel growth around cancer	Avastin	Experimental
Herbal/dietary	Supports nutrition and immune system in patient	Experimental	Experimental

Immunotherapy

Immunotherapy remains the subject of much research. New agents and approaches that work by promoting activation of the immune system continue to be studied. I will focus on two immunotherapies, monoclonal antibodies and non-specific agents, that stimulate the immune system but may also work through non-immune system mechanisms.

Monoclonal Antibodies

Antibodies are proteins that are made from B cells after exposure to an infectious organism. Each antibody is unique: An antibody that binds to a portion of a Salmonella bacterium, for example, cannot bind to any other bacteria. This specificity is how the immune system can carefully eliminate a particular bacterium. The antibody binds to the bacteria and attracts other immune system elements to get rid of it. Immunologists have studied this process in depth. They were determined to make antibodies for targeting other molecules, which turned out to be one of the most important discoveries in biology!

Monoclonal antibodies are specially designed to target almost any molecule. A variety of approaches using monoclonal antibodies for cancer therapy with several antibodies are now approved by the FDA for the treatment of B-cell malignancies and breast cancer. The potency of monoclonal antibodies may also be increased by linking cellular toxins or radioisotopes to the antibodies, which improves local killing of targeted tumor cells.

Because initial antibody production was done in animals, the antibody was recognized as a foreign protein in humans. A strong immune response against the antibody destroyed it before it could do its job. This issue has been dealt with by generating "humanized" antibodies that are not rejected by the immune system. Most of the current monoclonal antibodies in clinical development are partially or completely humanized.

Monoclonal antibodies can also be directed against growth factors or other signaling molecules on the surface of tumor cells inducing cell death. This has already shown promise in treating breast cancer and B-cell lymphoma. HER-2/neu is a receptor found on the surface of many breast cancer cells. A humanized monoclonal antibody that targets HER-2/neu, called Herceptin, was generated, and has shown promise when used in combination with chemotherapy for the treatment of breast cancer. Similarly, B cells have a cell-surface molecule called CD20. An antibody, Rituxan, has been developed that seems effective against B-cell lymphomas. The success of these monoclonal antibodies suggests that this general approach may be helpful in other types of cancer as well. The monoclonal antibody cetuximab (Erbitux®), which targets the epidermal growth factor receptor on cancer cells, has been approved by the FDA for the treatment of advanced colon cancer.

Other strategies using monoclonal antibodies have been developed. A number of large complex molecules called gangliosides are found on the surface of melanoma cells. Monoclonal antibodies have been generated against many of these gangliosides, with mixed results in early clinical trials. In other experiments, a number of specific toxins, such as radioactive isotopes, bacterial toxins, and chemotherapy agents, have been added to monoclonal antibodies.

Thalidomide

The drug thalidomide (Thalomid®) was used as a sleeping pill and to prevent morning sickness during pregnancy in the 1950s, until the drug was found to cause birth defects, stunting the growth of the arms and legs in infants. It was banned in the 1960s. Interest in thalidomide continued, however, because it appeared to alleviate some leprosy symptoms. Recently, we've had a glimmer that thalidomide may be useful for the treatment of cancer.

Thalidomide is an anti-inflammatory agent and blocks the release of certain inflammatory cytokines. Thalidomide can also stimulate T cells, suggesting that it may have profound effects on the immune system. In addition, thalidomide inhibits angiogenesis, the process of new blood vessel growth, which is helpful in fighting cancer. According to some studies, thalidomide may even directly inhibit the growth of cancer cells. Several clinical trials of thalidomide have been done, with beneficial effects seen in a type of cancer called multiple myeloma. Thalidomide is now being studied in melanoma, especially in combination with other chemotherapy drugs. The results of larger randomized studies are needed before the role of thalidomide can be fully evaluated.

Thalidomide is an oral drug and can be easily administered at home.

Because of the risk of birth defects it cannot be used in anyone who is pregnant. The medication must also be kept away from anyone who might become pregnant, since even a single dose can induce birth defects. Typically you must take a pregnancy test before considering thalidomide and must agree to avoid pregnancy by not having sex, or using an effective form of birth control. Thalidomide can also not be used if you are nursing a baby. Men must also avoid unprotected sex if they are taking thalidomide. The dose of thalidomide varies, depending on the clinical study, and should be discussed carefully with your doctor.

The main side effect of thalidomide is drowsiness, and so you should avoid alcohol intake or operating automobiles or other machinery. I often prescribe a lower dose and then increase the dose gradually over a period of several weeks to avoid the fatigue associated with thalidomide. Another way to avoid drowsiness is to take the medication at night just before bed, although usually we spread the doses out through the day. The other main side effect is constipation, which can often be prevented by using stool softeners and fiber supplements before taking the drug.

Other side effects are less common and include damage to the peripheral nerves located in the hands and feet. This may feel like burning, numbness, or tingling in the arms, hands, legs, or feet. If this occurs, it is usually necessary to stop taking thalidomide, but this is a decision that must be made in consultation with your doctor. Other less common side effects include skin rash, fever, headache, rapid heart rate, low blood pressure, swelling of the face and legs, dry mouth, nausea, increased appetite, mood changes, irregular menstrual period, low white blood cell count, thyroid problems, and problems with blood sugar levels.

Based on the variety of different effects observed with thalidomide researchers are designing new thalidomide derivatives. These drugs are being tested and developed to specifically act as T-cell stimulants or inhibitors of blood vessel growth. These agents are just starting to be tested in the clinic for a variety of cancers, including melanoma. Further research is needed to optimize the role of thalidomide and its derivatives in the treatment of melanoma.

Targeted Therapy

The close scrutiny of the genome in cancer cells has yielded a large number of new targets for drug development. The genetic instability inherent to cancer cells results in many gene mutations. Some of these mutations produce proteins that become overly active and promote the survival of the cancer cell. In cancer the continued signal to grow and divide is not normal. A new class of drugs targets these abnormally active proteins and the pathways that deliver survival signals to the cell. Whereas monoclonal antibodies are useful for targeting large proteins, such as those on the surface of the cell, smaller molecules may be able to enter the cell and block proteins that are overactive inside the cell. This approach has led to several exciting discoveries over the past few years, including FDA approval of new agents for other cancers. The next few years will witness even more new drugs for clinical testing and usher in a new era in cancer therapy.

The use of targeted inhibitors of signal pathways has shown much promise, but we've now uncovered a serious problem with the general strategy. While blocking one pathway or protein may be helpful for a time, exposure to such drugs may lead to new pathways taking over the functions of the blocked pathway. This so-called "resistance" can be compared to the resistance that occurs after using certain antibiotics for prolonged periods. Clever bacteria eventually evolve into organisms that can resist the antibiotic and grow right through them. Cancer cells may do the same thing when blocked by targeted therapy. Nonetheless, this approach may be especially useful when combined with other drugs; it may be necessary to block multiple pathways or proteins to more effectively prevent cancer cells from surviving.

I want to focus on two such new, targeted drugs. One has been well established and FDA approved for leukemia and a rare type of sarcoma, and the other is just starting clinical testing and is being tested in melanoma.

Gleevec

One set of proteins that are often overly active in cancer cells are called protein kinases. An inhibitor of multiple protein kinases is called imatinib (Gleevec®). The protein kinases are especially active in a type of leukemia called chronic myeloid leukemia (CML), so Gleevec was first tested in patients with CML. Several clinical trials demonstrated significant responses in CML patients, as well as a benefit in survival, and suggested that some patients could actually be cured of the disease. The FDA approved Gleevec for CML in 2001. Resistance may become a problem for those patients receiving Gleevec as single-agent therapy.

Gastrointestinal stromal tumors (GIST) are a rare type of cancer that occurs in about 5,000 patients every year in the United States. The tumors occur in the stomach and gastrointestinal tract. The cells giving rise to GIST tumors over-express certain protein kinases that can be blocked by Gleevec. Studies in patients with GIST demonstrated reduction of the cancers and suggested that Gleevec is an effective treatment in randomized clinical trials. This resulted in FDA approval of Gleevec for GIST tumors.

Some of the same protein kinases active in CML and GIST tumors may also be active in melanoma cells, but clinical studies have not shown Gleevec a benefit for melanoma yet.

Gleevec is available as a pill and can be taken at home. The common side effects of Gleevec include fluid retention, nausea, vomiting, diarrhea, skin rash, muscle cramps, liver toxicity, and lower blood cell counts. Typically, these side effects are mild.

Raf Kinase Inhibitors

The BRAF gene encodes a protein kinase that differs from those targeted by Gleevec. In studies using advanced genome screening of melanoma cells, mutations in the BRAF gene were identified in a majority of melanoma cells tested. The Raf pathway that leads to signaling keeps melanoma cells alive, and so blocking this pathway has become a focus for new drug development. Recently a new agent that blocks BRAF, one member of the Raf pathway, has been developed and has started clinical testing in patients with melanoma. Early studies suggested some benefit with this drug when combined with chemotherapy treatment in melanoma patients.

In the future, researchers will likely identify new kinases and other proteins involved in melanoma cell survival. Drugs that block these signal pathways will be developed and must be tested in well-designed clinical trials. The possibility of combining targeted drugs with chemotherapy, immunotherapy, or other treatment agents also awaits clinical investigation.

Gene Therapy

Once we understood that there are many genetic defects in cancer cells and that we can manipulate genes, it was logical to think that abnormal genes could be turned off in cancer cells. Similarly, some cancer cells may be missing good genes that work to turn off the cancer process. Gene therapy is a new field that either turns off abnormal genes or brings a new gene into a cancer cell that lacks it.

Strictly speaking, gene therapy refers to the introduction of genetic material into humans, usually resulting in the modification of specific cells. Table 14-2 lists some of the general strategies that use gene therapy for cancer. The advances in genome sequencing have led to a large number of genes for targeting in cancer cells. A great deal of research has focused on how to deliver new genes into cancer cells. At present this remains a major obstacle to successful gene therapy. Currently, genes are usually inserted into cancer cells through the injection of vectors, or agents that are used to deliver new genes into target cells. The most commonly used vectors are viruses, although there are new efforts to identify other vectors for gene delivery.

Table 14-2. General strategies for gene therapy

Strategy	Example
Reversal of abnormal gene function	Anti-sense gene silencing
Replacement of missing genes	Insertion of tumor suppressor gene
Enhanced chemosensitivity	Thymidine kinase/gancyclovir treatment
Tumor immunotherapy	Insertion of genes that promote immune responses

In gene therapy, first the DNA encoding the gene must get to the target cell, in most cases the cancer cell. Once the gene arrives it must enter the cancer cell, make its way to the nucleus of the cell where DNA is stored, and begin to produce the protein encoded by the gene. The ideal method for delivering genes into this complex process has not been discovered, despite intense research. Table 14-3 lists some of the methods that have been tried. Most efforts have used viruses since these naturally seek out cells and enter them. Many viruses actually make their way to the nucleus of the cell and so seem like a perfect way to get genes into the cell. Obviously, when viruses are used, the danger is that the virus itself may cause serious injury. Therefore, specialized viruses—those that are less harmful to people but can still enter cells and deliver genes to the nucleus—are used.

Table 14-3. Vectors for gene therapy

Classification	Vector
Viruses	Retrovirus
	Adenovirus
	Adeno-associated virus

Classification	Vector
Molecules	Poxviruses
	Herpes viruses
	DNA
	RNA
	Protein
	Peptides
Whole cells	Cancer cells
	T cells
	Dendritic cells

While viruses are a logical way to bring genetic information into cells, it is possible to directly inject DNA. Specialized carriers are necessary to make sure that the DNA survives in the body and enters the desired cells. This is a significant problem with DNA. Since the ultimate outcome of DNA delivery is to produce a protein that functions in the cell, proteins or fragments of proteins called peptides can be injected. Thus far, it has been difficult to get these small molecules into the appropriate cells. These synthetic molecules are easier to develop and use than live viruses. Non-viral methods of gene delivery have no risk of infection, no size limitations, and can be made in the laboratory. However, these molecules are not very efficient at getting into cells and may not last long enough.

In its simplest form, gene therapy can insert a gene that is missing from a cancer cell. When replaced into the cell, genes may stop the cancer process. Called tumor-suppressor genes, they can be placed into any vector for delivery to the cancer cells.

A number of strategies have been used to increase the immune response against cancer, particularly for melanoma. This includes delivering agents to melanoma cells that may make them more immunogenic, or likely to be targeted by the immune system. My own research has used poxviruses for bringing molecules into melanoma cells to increase their ability to activate T cells. Other immunotherapy approaches have utilized gene therapy modified tumor cells as vaccines. For example, cytokines such as GM-CSF can be inserted into tumor cells, which then are killed and used as powerful vaccines. Similarly, T cells and dendritic cells can be modified by gene therapy and then transferred into patients.

Although animal models have documented the benefits of gene therapy, clinical trials have only just started and must be completed before the role of gene therapy can be fully defined. Future progress in gene therapy will depend on developing better vectors, new strategies, combination treatments, and the results of clinical trials.

Anti-Angiogenesis

Cancer cells require the growth of specialized blood vessels to bring them nutrients to stay alive. A large amount of research has been done to try and understand how and why these blood vessels grow and has led to a variety of drugs that block their growth. When the blood vessels are disrupted, the cancer cells cannot get their nutrients and will die. This strategy works well in laboratory animals, and now evidence shows that it also works when combined with chemotherapy in patients with colon cancer.

The process of forming and maintaining these new blood vessels, called angiogenesis, is highly regulated and complex. One family of proteins, among several others, is called vascular endothelial growth factor (VEGF) and is known to promote blood vessel growth. New blood vessel growth begins when VEGF binds to a receptor on the surface of existing blood vessel cells, called endothelial cells. What causes the release of these angiogenic factors in the first place? There is increasing evidence that the trigger may be a low oxygen level that occurs as cancers grow larger. In order to continue their growth they require new blood vessels to bring in more oxygen. The point at which this occurs has been referred to as the **angiogenic switch.** VEGF appears to be important in all aspects of this complex process.

A number of new treatment options have been developed, based on a better understanding of the angiogenic process. Among the most promising new agents have been monoclonal antibodies targeted to VEGF. These antibodies prevent VEGF from triggering its receptor on the blood vessels, which in turn stops the cancer from getting its oxygen and nutrients. In preliminary clinical studies this therapy has been safe and makes tumors regress in many cases. Recently, the FDA approved one such monoclonal antibody called bevacizumab (Avastin®) when given with chemotherapy for patients with advanced colon cancer. This encouraging event should spur continued research into other anti-angiogenesis agents.

Complementary and Alternative Medicine

Complementary and alternative medicine (CAM) is a relatively new field of research that seeks to study the effects of non-traditional approaches on health and cancer treatment. Alternative medicine refers to practices that are used in place of traditional therapy: for example, when a patient decides to use herbal supplements rather than have chemotherapy for cancer. Complementary medicine refers to practices that are used to complement traditional treatment, such as using a special diet in combination with immunotherapy for melanoma. Although the use of special diets and herbs is most effective when used long before cancer exists in the body, the application of alternative medicine to melanoma and other cancers is still worth considering. Although little scientific evidence that alternative medicine is effective in treating melanoma has been established, when used in tandem with standard treatment, many patients may stand to benefit.

Patient safety and the possibility of making a disease worse needs to be considered when thinking about any alternative medicine strategy. In order to better evaluate new claims and document the safety of various alternative medicine approaches, the National Institutes of Health has established the National Center for Complementary and Alternative Medicine to evaluate the role of alternative medicine in traditional health care. While this is a welcome development, keep in mind that most alternative medicine approaches are not regulated as strictly as pharmaceutical agents. Therefore, it is important to make decisions about pursuing alternative and complementary medicine techniques with your doctor and to be sure that they will not interfere with any scheduled traditional therapy.

The National Center for Complementary and Alternative Medicine recognizes five general categories of alternative medicine (see Table 14-4). **Alternative medical systems** are based on principles and theories espoused in many non-Western cultures. These approaches include homeopathic medicine, naturopathic medicine, traditional Chinese medicine, and Ayurveda. **Mind-body intervention** refers to methods that enhance the mind's influence over bodily function and symptoms: patient support groups, meditation, prayer, music therapy, and cognitive-behavioral therapy. **Biological/diet-based therapies** utilize natural substances found in nature, such as organic foods, vitamins, and herbal supplements. **Manipulative and body-based methods** use movement of the body or its parts to relax or alleviate specific symptoms and include body massage, chiropractic, and osteopathic procedures. **Energy therapies** use electromagnetic or biologic fields for therapeutic purposes. Although such energy fields are not known to exist or mediate any health effects thus far, some forms of therapeutic touch may be helpful and similar to massage therapy.

Actually, many of my patients have a keen interest in using alternative medicine approaches. I always explain that some of the strategies may be worth pursuing, as we do not have solid evidence for or against certain claims. I urge caution in selecting alternative approaches and advise common sense. Taking a multi-vitamin tablet once a day when trying to build up the immune system during immunotherapy treatment, for example, is quite appropriate. On the other hand, it is unwise to try unknown herbal preparations in the middle of chemotherapy. The safety of many supplements is not consistent and may change from time to time, which leads to inequalities in response and additional safety concerns. Consultation with a nutritionist or expert in complementary medicine approaches is available at our center for interested patients. I caution my patients that these approaches do not *cure* melanoma. Nevertheless we can develop a plan to provide not only state-of-the-art conventional therapy, but also complementary medicine techniques that promote relaxation, reduce stress, and engender a general state of well-being.

Table 14-4. Types of alternative and complementary medicine approaches

Category	Approach	Comments	Indications
Alternative Medical Systems	Acupuncture	Ancient Chinese approach using thin needles	Pain relief
	Ayurveda	Ancient Indian technique uses diet and herbs	Promotes general well being; useful for prevention of disease
	Homeopathic medicine	Uses small quantities of medicine to cure symptoms caused by the same medicine in large doses	Uncertain benefit
	Naturopathic medicine	System based on healing power in the body; uses nutrition and lifestyle changes	Uncertain benefit

Category	Approach	Comments	Indications
	Traditional chinese medicine	Balances emotional, spiritual, mental, and physical needs through diet, exercise, and meditation	Promotes general well being
	Qi gong	Part of Chinese medicine combining movement, meditation, and breathing	Improves energy and immune function
	Reiki	Japanese technique uses healer's touch to alleviate symptoms	Pain relief and general well being
Mind-Body Interventions	Aromatherapy	Essential oils used to promote health	Alleviates side effects of chemotherapy
Biological/Diet Based Therapies	Dietary supplements	Includes vitamins, herbs, enzymes, metabolites, and organ tissue (i.e., shark cartilage)	Important for disease prevention
Manipulative and Body-based Methods	Chiropractic medicine	Based on the relationship between body structure and function	Pain relief
	Osteopathic medicine	Conventional approach based on belief that body systems work together and disturbance in one organ affects others	Pain relief; restores function and general well being
	Massage therapy	Manipulates muscles and soft tissue	Promotes relaxation and general well being

Category	Approach	Comments	Indications
Energy Therapies	Electromagnetic fields	Invisible force that surrounds electrical devices and the Earth	Unproven benefit
	Therapeutic touch	Healing force of the therapist affects patients	Promotes relaxation and well being

All of the treatments discussed in Chapters 12–14 depend on clinical trials to determine just how effective these new agents will be for patients with melanoma. In the next chapter, I examine clinical trials in depth.

Columbia Melanoma Center Case Studies

Roberto is a fifty-five-year-old who discovered a dark mole on his scalp, which began to grow. A biopsy revealed malignant melanoma, and he underwent wide local excision. He was well for two years, when a routine chest scan revealed multiple lung nodules. A biopsy confirmed that the melanoma had spread to the lungs. He was treated with chemotherapy, but did not respond and was referred to the Melanoma Center. We discussed the options and decided to treat him with high-dose interleukin-2 (IL-2). He tolerated the treatment well and had a partial response with a 50 percent reduction in the size of his lung melanoma. However, four months after completing IL-2 he complained of a headache and an MRI of the brain showed a new brain melanoma lesion. This was treated with gamma knife radiation and he recovered. Following treatment of his brain melanoma he asked about participating in an experimental clinical trial. He decided to enter a study testing Gleevec and was enrolled in the study for six months. He continues to feel well and has not had recurrence of his melanoma or growth of the melanoma in the lung.

Ask Your Doctor

If you are interested in targeted therapy or complementary treatment, ask the following questions:

1. *Do you have any new studies using innovative strategies?* These drugs are only available through clinical trials and change all the time. You should ask your doctor about which trials may be available and which you would qualify for. If there are no studies, you can search for potential clinical trials through the National Cancer Institute (www.nci.nih.gov). Some studies may exclude patients if they have had prior therapy so it is important to prioritize the order of treatment. This depends on how rapidly the disease is progressing and the availability of other standard treatment options. In general, it is best to start with standard therapy and move to experimental treatments when standard options fail.

2. *Should I consider complementary medicine?* Some forms of alternative and complementary medicine may help alleviate pain, provide relaxation, and promote general well-being. However, this is not a substitute for standard treatment. You can ask to meet with experts in complementary medicine and consider integrating some techniques with your standard therapy. If you do decide to take herbs or begin a new diet, you should inform your doctor, since unexpected interactions with standard drugs may occur.

3. *Should I be referred to a melanoma center?* If your doctor does not have access to new targeted agents, you may ask to be referred to a larger melanoma center where such treatment may be available.

CHAPTER FIFTEEN

What are Clinical Trials?

CLINICAL RESEARCH IS an area of medical investigation that evaluates new medications and treatment regimens for patients with diseases such as melanoma. Clinical research is experimental but most clinical investigators are now rigorously trained and they conduct research under the most stringent ethical and moral guidelines. Furthermore, an increasing number of regulatory agencies and committees review any clinical research proposal to make sure that the scientific principles are sound, that patients are protected from any harm, that meaningful information will be obtained, and that all results, good and bad, are reported. The approval of all new drugs in medicine is from appropriately designed clinical research.

As a melanoma specialist, I often advise patients to enter a clinical research trial. There is never a guarantee of a benefit, although many clinical research studies are based on the best laboratory research aimed at finding new drugs or vaccines for melanoma. Just as there is no guarantee of a benefit, there may also be no guarantee that the treatment will not be harmful. Some studies are designed to determine the side effects of new drugs, and certain patients may have atypical responses even if other patients are fine. Nevertheless, most new drugs are heavily tested in animals before being tested in patients, so the safety profile is often, but not always, predictable. If there is no guarantee of benefit or safety, why should you consider a clinical trial? The answer that I most commonly give to my patients is that, despite these drawbacks, some patients, after all else has failed, will respond to treatment. I think an even more compelling reason is that participation in clinical research helps all future patients with melanoma. I am impressed by how important this reason is for so many of my patients. The only way to determine if new agents work against melanoma is through clinical research; each patient can make a big difference in the hunt for a cure by participating.

Types of Clinical Research Trials

Clinical trials are based on a number of scientific, medical, economic, and statistical methods that allow clinical investigators to evaluate new treatment regimens or interventions for specific diseases. There are many different types of clinical trials (see Table 15-1). Your doctor may choose to be an investigator on a clinical trial or may refer you to another doctor who has a clinical trial. There may be a clinical trial for different aspects of a disease, including trials for patients with active disease, successfully treated disease, or at high risk of disease recurrence.

The most common type of clinical trial is a **therapeutic** or treatment trial. A therapeutic trial evaluates the benefits of a new drug, combination of drugs, or other therapeutic intervention, such as a new surgical procedure or type of radiation therapy. Therapeutic trials are appropriate for melanoma patients who have not responded to other treatments, or who may be unable or unwilling to have standard therapy. All therapeutic trials are approved by the United States Food and Drug Administration (FDA) as well as local review committees. Most therapeutic trials are based on evidence that a drug or treatment has shown some effect in treating melanoma in the laboratory or in animal models. In some cases, new drugs that have been effective against other types of cancer may also be tested in melanoma. In general, patients must have melanoma in order to participate in a therapeutic trial.

Another type of clinical trial, called a **prevention trial,** is designed to prevent melanoma from occurring. **Prevention trials** differ in that patients do not have melanoma when participating in these studies. In some cases, prevention trials attempt to prevent melanoma in high-risk patients: patients with a strong family history of melanoma in several close relatives or those with dysplastic nevus syndrome, for example. Other prevention studies are for patients who have had a melanoma treated and aim at preventing a recurrence. Prevention trials have been very successful in other diseases, including breast cancer and colon cancer, although few are focused on melanoma as of this writing.

A **screening trial** tries to find new methods of detecting cancer in people. Early detection allows earlier treatment and usually improves the outcome. Screening trials of skin evaluation by dermatologists suggested that this method did result in earlier detection of melanoma and may improve the survival rate for patients who are at risk for developing melanoma. Based on such screening studies we now recommend annual skin screening for patients at risk.

Unfortunately, many treatments for melanoma and other cancers are often accompanied by severe side effects. Therefore, it is important to include measures of the quality of a patient's life when undergoing individual treatments. A **quality of life** trial tests the quality of life for specific interventions. Occasionally, quality of life is included in a therapeutic or prevention trial. This study usually involves measuring general well being through a questionnaire or by an interview with a health care professional. The information obtained from these trials is important for better understanding the effects of treatments on all aspects of a patient's life.

The last kind of clinical trial is a **laboratory correlative trial.** This trial does not include a treatment or prevention regimen, but simply collects blood or tissue from patients. The collected specimens are used for analysis of genes, proteins, or immune responses. This has become especially important over the past few years with advances in genetics, molecular biology, and immunology. These trials are often used to identify new drug targets, predict responses to treatment, determine prognostic outcome based on molecular patterns, and evaluate immune responses. Many times a laboratory correlative trial is incorporated into a therapeutic or prevention trial.

Table 15-1. Clinical trials categories

Trial Design
Therapeutic trial
Prevention trial
Screening trial
Quality of life trial
Laboratory correlative trial

Trial Phase
I (safety and dosing)
II (effectiveness)
III (comparison to current standard of care)

Trial Sponsor
Investigator-initiated
Industry sponsored
Cooperative group
Government-sponsored

Phases of Clinical Trials

Clinical trials are conducted in specific phases to collect different types of information. This point is often not well understood. The phase of a clinical trial does not indicate the effectiveness of the drug or agent, but rather defines the scientific goal of the clinical trial. Once a new drug, vaccine, or procedure is identified that may have an impact against disease the agent is tested in a Phase I clinical trial. The Phase I clinical trial is the first time the agent is given to patients. The goal of a Phase I trial is to determine how much drug can be safely given to patients. Another goal is to evaluate the side effects that occur with the new agent. Phase I trials are typically very small since the dose and side effect profile can be obtained quickly. When I conduct a Phase I clinical trial, I include approximately ten–twenty patients. Sometimes patients may respond well to the agent, which encourages us to proceed with testing the new drug. However, Phase I trials are not designed to determine if the drug or agent is effective, because there are too few participants. These studies are important, since larger studies would be more difficult if the dose of drug or the type of side effects were not known.

In Phase II clinical trials, the goal is to determine if the new drug, vaccine, or procedure has an effect on the disease. These trials test the new agent in a group of patients, typically fifty to one hundred, with similar disease characteristics—for example, patients with Stage IV melanoma. The dose of drug used is determined from the Phase I clinical trial and all patients in the Phase II trial receive the same dose of medication. The Phase II clinical trial gives us information for therapeutic trials about how effective the new approach is in treating the disease, or preventing the disease in prevention trials. For most Phase I and II clinical trials all patients receive the new agent. Some Phase II trials test combinations of new drugs with established treatment strategies to see if there is a better outcome in patients given both therapies.

If an experimental drug, vaccine, or procedure shows an adequate safety profile and evidence of clinical effects in Phase I and II clinical trials, a Phase III clinical trial may be conducted. The Phase III trial is used to compare the experimental treatment to whatever the standard of care is for the disease being evaluated. These studies are conducted on a larger number of patients, usually one hundred to one thousand, depending on the expected outcomes. In Phase III clinical trials patients are usually divided into two groups. One group receives the new experimental agent and is referred to as the treatment group. The other group receives the current standard of care and is called the control group.

Patients are selected for the two groups in a process called randomization, much like flipping a coin, that is often done by a computer. If there is no standard or if eligible patients have already received the standard, a placebo may be used. A placebo is a drug or treatment that looks like the experimental drug or treatment but contains no drug. Placebo is commonly used when there is no effective treatment. This study design allows investigators to compare the experimental treatment to the standard of care. The FDA also uses the results of these studies to decide if new drugs or treatments actually improve the outcome for patients. Phase III clinical trials are very important, since they are the only way to know if a new drug is truly helpful. It is vital to have patients willing to participate in such trials.

Clinical Trial Sponsorship

Clinical trials may be sponsored by different sources. A sponsor is the person or group responsible for the clinical trial design and its financial support. No particular type of sponsor is better or worse than another, so this information need not be taken into consideration. Clinical trials based on a clinical investigator's own research are called **investigator-initiated trials** and are often supported by research grants from the government or industry. Many clinical trials originate from pharmaceutical or biotechnology companies and are referred to as **industry-sponsored trials.** They are supported by the company developing the new drug or agent; the company usually supplies the drug and other expenses to cover the costs of the clinical trial. In the United States, Canada, and Europe, several cooperative oncology groups composed of many different medical centers and hospitals have formed to develop clinical trials for patients with cancer. Although the names were based on the location of the original participating institutions or the original goals of the group, nearly all of the groups now focus on a variety of cancers. The cooperative groups include many of the top physicians and scientists involved in cancer research. The groups meet regularly to discuss the most promising new drugs or approaches and develop their own clinical trials based on mutual agreement that the trials represent the most important drugs and strategies to test. These clinical trials are referred to as **cooperative group trials.** Table 15-2 lists some of the cooperative groups and their contact information. Many clinical trials supported by the cooperative groups are available to all oncologists through the efforts of the National Cancer Institute.

Table 15-2. National oncology cooperative groups

Cooperative Group	Main Focus	Headquarters	Web site
Eastern Cooperative Oncology Group (ECOG)	Most cancers, including melanoma	Boston, MA	www.ecog.org
Southwest Oncology Group (SWOG)	Most cancers, including melanoma	San Antonio, TX	www.swog.org
Cancer and Leukemia Group B (CALGB)	Most cancers, including melanoma	Chicago, IL	www.calgb.org
American College of Surgeons Oncology Group (ACOSOG)	Surgical approaches for cancer	Chicago, IL	www.facs.org
North Central Cancer Treatment Group (NCCTG)	Most cancers	Rochester, MN	http://ncctg.mayo.edu
National Surgical Adjuvant Breast and Bowel Project (NSABP)	Breast and colon cancer	Pittsburgh, PA	www.nsabp.pitt.edu
Gynecologic Oncology Group (GOG)	Gynecologic cancers	Philadelphia, PA	www.gog.org
Children's Oncology Group (COG)	Pediatric cancers	Arcadia, CA	www.childrensoncology group.org

Cooperative Group	Main Focus	Headquarters	Website
Radiation Therapy Oncology Group (RTOG)	Radiation treatments for cancer	Philadelphia, PA	www.rtog.org
European Organization for Research and Treatment of Cancer (EORTC)	Most cancers	Brussels, Belgium	www.eortc.be

Eligibility for Clinical Trials

All clinical trials have eligibility criteria, usually based on selecting patients who are most likely to benefit from treatment. Other considerations include the ability of patients to tolerate treatment, the probability that the patient will stay alive for the duration of the clinical trial, and whether the patient needs to receive standard treatment. The trial eligibility defines the type of cancer and stage of disease for patients. For example, some studies may only be open to those with Stage IV melanoma, while others may only allow Stage III melanoma patients to participate. Similarly, some clinical trials will accept only cutaneous melanoma patients, and others will also allow those with mucosal melanoma or ocular melanoma to participate. The presence of brain metastases is often an exclusion from participation, because patients with melanoma in the brain require immediate intervention. Many studies will allow patients who have completed treatment for brain melanoma to participate in a study.

Most clinical trial eligibility also requires a careful medical screening to make sure that there are no serious medical conditions—other than cancer—that might prevent administration of the treatment or cause more side effects. The screening consists of a medical history and physical examination, X-ray tests, EKG, and blood and urine tests. Some studies will also require an HIV test because patients with HIV may be at increased risk for complications, as, for example, when a live virus vaccine is being used. Some clinical trials may also have other requirements based on how the drug or agent is thought to work.

Many clinical trials are also designed for patients who are at a particular point in their treatment. Some studies require that previous standard treatment has been given and failed. The rationale for this is that patients first should be able to try the best standard of care, such as Interleukin-2 for Stage IV melanoma. If this fails then they become eligible for a clinical trial. However, some studies require that patients have had no previous therapy. The rationale is that prior treatment may interfere with the benefit of the new experimental drug. For example, if patients have had chemotherapy it may be difficult to get a vaccine to work properly. In these cases, patients may decide to enter the clinical trial first and receive a vaccine with few expected side effects. If the experimental vaccine does not work, then the patient can start standard chemotherapy. These decisions can be complex and should be made in consultation with your doctor.

Patients who participate in a clinical trial are usually required to have a baseline CT scan of their disease sites for Stage IV melanoma or to prove there is no disease for other stages. In addition, blood tests and other studies may be required. In order to have the most consistent population of patients these studies must usually be completed within a few weeks of the trial's start date. Most clinical trials do not allow other treatment while under study to avoid unexpected interactions between experimental agents and other drugs. If you are in a clinical trial, report any new medications or treatments to your doctor before using them.

Although this may all seem very complicated and may require seemingly unnecessary tests, a major advantage of participating in clinical trials is that you will receive a lot of attention. Such vigilance means your doctor knows what is going on, may detect changes early, and be able to switch you to other therapies. In the best case scenario, you may also show evidence of good response to a new treatment. In any event, when you are applying for a clinical trial, your medical record will be reviewed carefully to make sure that you meet all eligibility requirements. Most of these criteria were designed to provide you with the most benefit and to make sure that the treatment is as safe as possible. If you do not qualify for one clinical trial you may qualify for another one. (See page 268 for finding clinical trials.)

Informed Consent

Before entering a clinical trial, you will have a discussion with the doctor responsible for the trial. During this meeting you will be told about the purpose of the clinical trial and why the investigator believes the treatment may be effective for melanoma. You will also be told about the procedures and tests required to determine if you are eligible. In addition, the type of treatment, doses, possible side effects, and other tests or procedures that may be done in conjunction with the experimental treatment will be discussed. The investigator should also tell you about alternative treatments to consider, including standard therapies. You will be told about the potential benefits, which may be completely unknown in a Phase I trial or fairly well established for a Phase III trial. You should be informed about how many patients are being recruited for the clinical trial and what costs, if any, you will need to pay for your participation. You will also be told when and why the clinical trial may be stopped. This typically occurs if your melanoma gets worse or if there are serious side effects. This information is listed in a document called an informed consent form. The form is approved at the hospital where the clinical trial is being conducted, by a committee called the institutional review board, or IRB. It has a contact phone number for the investigator and the IRB in case you need more information. Before you can start on a clinical trial you must sign the consent form. It gives the investigator permission to treat you as outlined in the form, although you can usually change your mind at any time. In my practice I like to give patients the consent form to review for at least a day or two so they can be sure to digest all the information. Many patients will have further questions after reading the consent form, and these questions should be answered before the form is signed. You should receive a copy of the signed consent form for your records.

In some cases you may be asked permission for your blood or body tissues to be used for other purposes. This is often found on a separate part of the consent form and requires a separate signature. For most investigators this is a very important and useful act for patients, since science and research is constantly changing. New laboratory techniques and methods are always being developed and the ability to store patient tissues is helpful in bringing new technology to the clinic. In most cases this does not result in direct benefit to a patient but does help the overall research effort in melanoma. Participation in blood and tissue collection can lead to new treatments that may help other patients with melanoma in the future.

Regulation of Clinical Research

The conduct of clinical research is a highly regulated process. Although there have been widely publicized deviations from the requirements, they are rare exceptions to the rule. Most clinical investigators are now required to undergo specialized training in the scientific and ethical conduct of research involving human subjects. Additionally, clinical trials are reviewed by numerous committees to make sure that they are appropriate before an investigator can test any new agent. Table 15-3 lists some of the committees that review our clinical protocols. This review process explains, in part, why it may take so long to get a new trial approved. The review is designed to keep patients safe and provide the most promising agents for treatment or prevention.

Table 15-3. Regulation of clinical trials

Review Committee or Agency	Review Goals
U.S. FDA	Approves all therapeutic trials for scientific rationale, study design, endpoints, and safety
Office of Biotechnology Activities, National Institutes of Health	Reviews all clinical trials involving recombinant DNA for safety issues
National Cancer Institute	Reviews and approves many clinical trials using NCI drugs, cooperative group studies, and government-funded clinical trials
Institutional Review Board (IRB)	Local hospital review board, which includes private citizens, that evaluates the logic of the trial and protection of subjects from harm
Cancer Center Committee	Committee at many large universities that provides additional review of scientific and statistical issues in melanoma trials; often required before IRB review
Institutional Biosafety Committee	Local hospital review board that determines any safety issues related to biologic or recombinant-DNA–containing agents
Data Safety Monitoring Board (DSMB)	Committee set up to evaluate the side effects and results of a clinical trial; group can recommend stopping a trial for safety reasons
Cooperative Group Committee	Reviews all clinical trials proposed in the cooperative group and prioritizes clinical trials

In addition to the regulatory reviews, strict rules for reporting all incidents and results of a clinical trial are enforced. Any side effects that are unexpected must be reported to all of the committees approving the clinical trial. Many clinical trials will also have a Data Safety Monitoring Board, or DSMB, established to monitor the clinical trial. This board usually is composed of professional and lay citizens who are not associated with the trial so that they can act in an objective and impartial manner. The board will review any side effects, and if there are too many incidents or if the treatment is more toxic than expected the DSMB may decide to stop the trial. In any event, all unexpected or severe side effects are reported to the IRB and FDA. Every clinical trial is also reviewed annually by the IRB, and a decision is made about whether to keep the study open based on the incidence of side effects, number of patients enrolled, and the effects of treatment.

Clinical trials also require expert review by biostatisticians, who help design the trial so that meaningful conclusions can be made. The biostatistician is an expert in the interpretation of numerical data and calculation of clinical outcomes. He or she is involved in every aspect of clinical trial design and helps determine how many patients are needed in the study, how to define the side effect profile, the effect on laboratory parameters, and how effective a treatment is for patients. Most, if not all of the committees listed in Table 15-3, include biostatisticians to help with these issues. Clinical trials also require data managers, experts in the collection and management of clinical data. This includes keeping careful records of the patient, prior treatment, results of blood and X-ray tests, amount of drug received, side effects observed, and information on how the patient responds to treatment. Most patients are seen on a regular follow-up basis to see how they are doing.

You can see that clinical trials require a great deal of manpower and are designed to be as safe as possible. Until other methods are developed, the clinical trial remains the only valid method for determining the effects of new drugs or treatments for patients with melanoma.

A Logical Order

Now that you know how clinical trials are organized and managed, how do you decide to enter a clinical trial? Which clinical trial should you choose? The answer depends on the stage of disease, the status of prior therapy, the availability of appropriate clinical trials, and the wishes of the patient. Some patients prefer to have standard treatment first and save clinical trials to try if standard therapy fails, whereas other patients may wish to start with a clinical trial. In general, I like to begin with standard therapy when it is available and effective. In the event that standard therapy does not work or is not possible, clinical trials should be considered.

It may require a bit of work to find an appropriate trial. Furthermore, at any given time clinical trials are at various stages, some being completed and others just getting started. Melanoma experts are aware of the current clinical trials for melanoma. I receive copies of medical records from patients all over the world to see if they are eligible for one of our clinical trials before they invest in travel or heightened expectations. Reviewing the medical record can often identify patients who are eligible or ineligible for specific trials. Since melanoma responds poorly to so many treatments, it may be necessary to try different trials before something works. Most physicians are willing to send patients to another doctor or center for a clinical trial.

Since some clinical trials exclude patients with prior therapy and others may require completion of standard treatment, clinical trials must be prioritized. For example, if there is a promising new treatment that is being tested only in patients with no other therapy this trial may be tried first. This can be followed by standard treatment if the clinical trial is not effective. Once standard treatment fails, patients can then be referred to a clinical trial that requires completion of standard therapy. Treatment decisions must be individualized. The goal is to develop a logical order for treatment. The decision about how to proceed should include the potential effectiveness of a particular experimental agent, the proximity of treatment to the patient, the eligibility requirements for the trial, and the preference of the patient.

How to Find Clinical Trials

If your doctor does not know of any clinical trials, you can find clinical trials on your own. In Appendix B is a list of melanoma resources that includes several Web sites that maintain a listing of currently active clinical trials for melanoma. The National Cancer Institute has one of the best sites and keeps a listing of melanoma clinical trials available throughout the country (800-4CANCER or www.nci.gov). Since extensive travel is often not feasible or possible for many patients, you can also contact a university medical center near your home. Many major medical centers have cancer centers or programs that support clinical research. These centers may have clinical trials or will be able to guide you to other centers that have such clinical trials.

Benefits and Drawbacks to Clinical Research

While there are many benefits from clinical trial participation, there are some drawbacks worth mentioning. Many clinical trials will require extra office visits, hospitalization, blood tests, and X-ray tests. This may prolong the time you are in the hospital or the doctor's office. In some cases, you may need to travel to medical centers farther from home and this can certainly be inconvenient. Although patients may benefit from a new drug, there is no guarantee and it is even possible that the side effects will be worse than anticipated. A major issue for many patients is the use of a placebo, which often is used in Phase III trials. In many cases you and your doctor will not know what you are receiving. These studies, called double blind studies, are important so that the real benefit of the treatment can be determined without bias by the patient or treating physician. This is a risk when participating in a clinical trial with a placebo, although many times this risk is worth taking. As mentioned, even if you are assigned to a placebo arm of a clinical trial you will receive all other care and attention, which may not be provided if you are not in a clinical trial. Many studies now limit placebo groups to one third, rather than one half of patients. In some cases, patients who receive placebo and do not respond will be able to receive the experimental drug. This is called a crossover study since the placebo patients can "cross over" to the experimental treatment. You should ask the investigator about the particulars of the placebo group if there is a placebo in the clinical trial you are considering.

In general, the benefits of clinical trials outweigh the drawbacks. Patients often have high expectations from clinical trials. There is never a guarantee that an experimental treatment will benefit an individual patient. However, most patients who agree to participate in a clinical trial will receive close attention and expert care. This usually provides patients with access to the best possible outcome. At the present time there are few effective options for patients with advanced stages of melanoma and fewer than 5 percent of all patients elect to participate in clinical trials. This may explain the slow rate of new drugs developed for melanoma over the past several years. A renewed commitment from scientists and industry to develop better drugs for melanoma is needed. An equal commitment from patients to participate in clinical trials is just as important. This joint effort will help identify new and more effective therapies for melanoma.

Columbia Melanoma Center Case Studies

Simon is a fifty-five-year-old man with a history of Stage III melanoma that was treated five years previously by a wide local excision of a left arm melanoma and a left axillary lymph node dissection. He recently noticed several new "nodules" over his right chest wall and a biopsy was consistent with metastatic melanoma. A CT scan of the chest revealed evidence of metastatic melanoma in the lungs. Simon went to his oncologist, who recommended chemotherapy. However, Simon and his wife were not happy with chemotherapy and requested that he be referred to a melanoma center for a clinical trial. Simon was referred to our center.

After reviewing his medical records and talking to Simon we decided that a clinical trial was possible. Simon agreed to participate in a clinical trial of a new vaccine treatment that was being developed as a Phase I investigator-initiated trial at our Melanoma Center. Simon underwent all of the blood tests, CT scans, and laboratory studies required for the clinical trial. He was treated with vaccine once a month for three months. Simon re-

ported no side effects except for some mild pain at the site of his vaccination. After three months his melanoma nodules disappeared and a CT
scan of the chest showed complete response of the melanoma in the
lungs. Simon agreed to give some extra blood and tissue samples, and
these were used to document that Simon had indeed developed an immune response against his melanoma. He remained free of melanoma for
one year but then noticed a new lump on his scalp. The lump was a
melanoma and this was treated by surgical excision. Thus far, there has
been no recurrence of melanoma at any other site and we continue to see
Simon every three months.

Although Simon had an initial good outcome with a complete response
to his melanoma, not every patient can expect this. However, this case represents what can happen when a patient decides to enter a clinical trial.
Even though he recurred about one year later, this melanoma was easily
treated by surgical excision. Simon is also followed very closely by our
team, and if the melanoma recurs again we have many options available
since he has not received any other treatment. Thus, for Simon the decision
to participate in a clinical trial was a good one.

Ask Your Doctor

If you are interested in clinical trials, ask the following questions:

1. *Am I a candidate for a clinical trial?* The first thing to do if interested
   in a clinical trial is to determine if you are eligible for the study. This
   will depend on the type of melanoma, stage of melanoma, your
   history of prior therapy, other medical conditions, blood tests, X-ray
   studies, and possibly other factors. Many of these factors can be
   found in your medical record and determined ahead of time. Other
   studies may be necessary before determining if you are eligible for a
   particular clinical trial. Your doctor or the principal investigator of the
   clinical trial can help determine which clinical trials you will be
   eligible for.

2. *What is the purpose of the clinical trial?* An important component of
   deciding whether to participate in a clinical trial is the scientific

rationale for the study. This is often based on animal studies or clinical trials of drugs in cancers other than melanoma. Those clinical trials with the most compelling scientific support should be considered first, especially when there are several trials available. Your doctor or a melanoma specialist can help explain how a particular drug or approach is thought to work and why it is a high or low priority.

3. *How long will the clinical trial take?* Most clinical trials will require that you have experimental treatment without receiving any other cancer therapies. It is important to know how long the treatment period will last since, if the experimental treatment does not work, you should be able to move on to the next treatment option. Since we typically obtain scans every three months, it is common for treatment periods to last three months or less. Any study that lasts longer should be questioned and you should be certain that scans can be obtained at three-month intervals to make sure that the melanoma is not getting worse despite the treatment provided on a clinical trial.

4. *What treatment is required for the clinical trial?* You should ask about what the treatment is, what dose will be used, and how the treatment will be given. For example, some medications may be in the form of a pill and others may require an intravenous injection in the hospital.

5. *Is there a placebo?* In Phase III clinical trials the experimental treatment is often compared to the best standard therapy or, when there is no effective standard treatment, a placebo. This information should be explained to you ahead of time so that you can make an informed decision about participating in a trial. In some cases you may be allowed to receive the experimental treatment if you are assigned to placebo. In some cases your doctor will know if you received placebo and in some cases your doctor will not know. This is all information that you should ask about before signing an informed consent form.

6. *What additional tests are required before or during the clinical trial?* Most clinical trials require additional tests, such as blood or urine

tests, EKG, X-rays, and occasionally other studies. You should ask about what additional studies are needed before starting and during the clinical trial. Some of these, such as CT scans, may be part of routine medical care but others may be additional tests. If they are not part of the normal care, insurance may not cover the costs of these tests.

7. *What are the side effects?* Although unexpected or unusual side effects are possible with any experimental therapy, there is often some sense of what side effects are possible. You should be told about what to expect, what some of the unexpected effects might be, and how these will be managed if they occur. You should understand whom to contact if such side effects occur. This usually requires that you contact the clinical study physician rather than your regular doctor.

8. *What alternatives are available?* You should be aware of other options that might be available for treatment. Then the options can be prioritized and you can have a logical order for treatment. This includes both other standard therapies, such as surgery, radiation, chemotherapy, immunotherapy, and experimental agents through clinical trials. It is important that participation in one study does not exclude you from treatment with other agents.

9. *What costs are associated with the study?* If tests or procedures are not routine they may not be covered by your regular health insurance. In many cases, these extra tests are covered by the study sponsor but you should ask about this before agreeing to participate in a clinical trial.

10. *How will my privacy be protected?* While there are now strict laws regulating the dissemination of health care information, when you participate in a clinical trial some of your health information will be shared with other groups, such as the FDA, IRB, or other committees that oversee clinical trials. In many states you will be required to sign another document that states you understand that this information will be made available for review by these regulatory bodies. In some cases the review agencies will not know your exact name but will

only review the medical information. This is essential for agencies and committees to evaluate the effectiveness of new treatments and to understand the side effects of new agents. In any event, most clinical investigators will be able to describe measures used to protect the confidentiality of subjects participating in their clinical trials.

11. *Who can I talk to about the clinical trial?* You should be given the name and phone number of the doctor responsible for the clinical trial. This individual or his/her designee should be able to answer any questions about the study and be available if there are any side effects or other complications during participation. In addition, there is often a research nurse available to deal with non-urgent medical problems and logistical issues. There should also be a contact from the hospital IRB who can answer questions about the clinical trial and an investigator if you have any concerns about the trial or its approval status.

12. *Can I change my mind about participating?* You can usually withdraw your consent for participation in a clinical trial at any time. However, this should be stated in writing in the informed consent form and you should certainly ask about this if there is any doubt.

13. *What reasons will be used to stop the clinical trial?* You should fully understand for what reasons an experimental treatment will be discontinued. Common reasons include the lack of response to a particular treatment, serious side effects in the patient, severe side effects in other patients, and decisions by companies to stop providing experimental agents. In the event that an experimental agent is approved by the FDA it may also be necessary to pay for continued access to the drug. This information can usually be found in the informed consent form.

14. *What if I respond to the treatment?* Hopefully you will have some type of beneficial response to an experimental agent. In this case, you should understand what will happen. Sometimes you will continue to be treated with the agent, but sometimes the agent will be stopped. In the event that the response is only partial, you should

be clear about whether treatment will continue or end. This is part of the design of a clinical trial and should be explained to you before starting the trial.

15. *What if I do not respond to the treatment?* In the event that you do not have a response to the agent used in a clinical trial, you will likely be removed from the study. You should have a backup plan ready, and this is where a logical order is important. If one study fails in your treatment, then a plan for another clinical trial or treatment with standard therapy should be ready to go. This way, no matter what happens, a logical progression through treatment options can proceed with minimal delays.

Conclusion

THE IDEA FOR writing *The Melanoma Book* came from a medical colleague, who urged me to share all the information I had accumulated on the subject of melanoma with patients everywhere. Only after I was working on the manuscript did I discover that my colleague was suffering from melanoma himself, lamenting that even *he* did not feel informed enough to make decisions about his treatment. Sadly, he died of his disease, one more reason I feel an urgency in getting this book to as many doctors and patients as possible.

I hope you have found all your questions answered in these pages, but equally important, I hope you will be inspired to participate in clinical trials. When melanoma patients decide to contribute time and effort to such research, they have the potential to help both themselves and those who are diagnosed later. Ultimately, it is through clinical trials that we will find a cure for melanoma. Until that day, I encourage you to seek the best possible treatment with the best qualified experts. It can make the difference between enduring melanoma and living with melanoma.

Appendix A: IL-2 Treatment Centers

The following centers in the United States have programs to treat melanoma patients with high-dose Interleukin-2 (IL-2):

Alabama

Birmingham
University of Alabama at
    Birmingham
    Robert Conry, MD
    205-978-0250

Florida

Gainesville
University of Miami Sylvester
    Cancer Center
    Lyn Feun, MD
    Pasquale Benedetto, MD
    305-243-4909

University of Florida Shands
    Medical Center
    Troy Guthrie, MD
    904-549-3072

Miami
The Mount Sinai Comprehensive
    Cancer Center

Jose Lutzky, MD
    305-535-3358

Tampa
Moffitt Cancer Center
    Adil Daud, MD
    813-972-8482
    Mayer Fishman, MD
    813-972-8400

Georgia

Atlanta
Emory University
    David Lawson, MD
    Wayne Harris, MD
    404-778-1900

Kentucky

Louisville
University of Louisville
    Damian Laber, MD
    Donald Miller, MD
    502-562-4370

Illinois
Chicago
Northwestern University
   Timothy M. Kuzel, MD
      312-695-0990

Rush-Presbyterian-St. Luke's
      Medical Center
   Kevin Conlon, MD
      312-942-5685

Indiana
Goshen
Goshen Center for Cancer Care
   Douglas Schwartzentruber, MD
      574-535-2888

Indianapolis
Indiana University
   Theodore Logan, MD
      317-274-3515

Maryland
Baltimore
Johns Hopkins University
   William Sharfman, MD
   Robert Pili, MD
      410-583-2970

Massachusetts
Boston
Beth Israel Deaconess Medical
      Center
   Michael Atkins, MD
   David McDermott, MD
      617-667-1936

Michigan
Ann Arbor
University of Michigan Cancer
      Center
   Bruce G. Redman, D.O.
      734-936-8906

Detroit
Wayne State University
   Lawrence E. Flaherty, MD
   Ulka Vaishampayan, MD
      313-745-9166

Minnesota
Minneapolis
University of Minnesota
   Arkadiusz Dudek, MD
      612-624-0123

New Hampshire
Hanover
Dartmouth-Hitchcock Medical
      Center
   Marc Ernstoff, MD
   Christopher P. Tretter, MD
      603-650-9464

New York
Buffalo
Roswell Park Cancer Institute
   Michael Wong, MD, PhD
      716-845-3516

New York City
Columbia University Medical
      Center

Howard L. Kaufman, MD
212-342-6042

North Carolina

Charlotte
Blumenthal Cancer Center
Richard White, MD
704-355-2884

Durham
Duke University
Jared Gollob, MD
919-668-3979

Ohio

Columbus
Ohio State University
Karie Kendra, MD
614-293-8619

Pennsylvania

Allentown
Saint Luke's Hospital
Lee Riley, MD, PhD
610-954-2140

Pittsburgh
University of Pittsburgh Cancer
Institute

Joseph Baar, MD
Sanjiv Agarwala, MD
412-648-6507

Tennessee

Nashville
Vanderbilt University Medical
Center
Jeff Sosman, MD
615-936-3831

Texas

Dallas
University of Texas Southwestern
Medical Center
Barry S. Levinson, MD
Barbara B. Haley, MD
214-648-7070

Houston
M.D. Anderson Cancer Center
Patrick Hwu, MD
713-745-7027

San Antonio
Southwest Texas Methodist
Hospital
Geoffrey Weiss, MD
210-567-4777

Appendix B: Melanoma Web sites

You can find additional information and resources on the treatment and prevention of melanoma at **www.TheMelanomaBook.com** as well as on the following Web sites:

Melanoma Education and Prevention

Alberta Society of Melanoma
www.melanoma.ca

American Academy of Dermatology, MelanomaNet
www.derm-infonet.com

American Association for Cancer Research
www.aacr.org

American Cancer Society
www.cancer.org

American Society of Clinical Oncology
www.asco.org

Center for Disease Control and Prevention, Melanoma Prevention
www.cdc.gov

The Eye Cancer Network
www.lafn.org/~bc534/ocularmelmets.htm

Interleukin-2 Patient Information
www.proleukin.com

Melanoma—The A,B,C's
www.melanoma.com/melanoma/index.jsp

The Melanoma Education Foundation
www.skincheck.com

Melanoma Patient's Information Page
www.mpip.org

The Melanoma Research Foundation
www.melanoma.org

National Center for Complementary and Alternative Medicine
nccam.nih.gov

The Skin Cancer Foundation
www.skincancer.org

Society for Melanoma Research
www.societymelanomaresearch.org

Specialized Centers for Melanoma Treatment

Columbia University Medical Center
www.columbiamelanomacenter.com

Dana Farber Cancer Institute
www.dfci.harvard.edu/pat/adult/treatment/diagnosis_page.asp?ref=dropdown
&type=adult&disease=melanoma

Dartmouth Medical Center
www.cancer.dartmouth.edu/melanoma/referral.shtml

Duke University
cancer.duke.edu/skin

Johns Hopkins University
www.hopkinskimmelcancercenter.org/specialtycenters/facility.cfm?facility
id=33

John Wayne Cancer Institute
www.jwci.org

H. Lee Moffit Cancer Center
www.moffitt.usf.edu/prevention_and_treatment/clinical_programs/cutane
ous/faqs.asp

M.D. Anderson Cancer Center
www.mdanderson.org/diseases/melanoma

Memorial Sloan Kettering Cancer Center
www.mskcc.org/mskcc/html/390.cfm

National Cancer Institute
www.nci.gov

Roswell Park Cancer Institute
www.roswellpark.org

University of California San Francisco
cc.ucsf.edu/clinical/melanoma.html

University of Michigan
www.cancer.med.umich.edu/learn/pwmelanoma.htm

University of Pennsylvania
www.penncancer.com/cancerprograms_detail.cfm?id=16

University of Pittsburgh
www.upci.upmc.edu/research/clinical/melanoma/index.html

University of Virginia
www.healthsystem.virginia.edu/internet/cancer/melanomades.cfm

Clinical Trials for Melanoma

American College of Surgeons Oncology Group
www.acosog.org

ClinicalTrials.gov
www.clinicaltrials.gov

Eastern Cooperative Oncology Group
www.ecog.org

Hospice Foundation of America
www.hospicefoundation.org

Melanoma Research Foundation
www.melanoma.org

National Cancer Institute
www.nci.nih.gov

New York City Melanoma Consortium
www.nycmelanomaconsortium.org

Radiation Therapy Oncology Group
www.rtog.org

Southwest Oncology Group
www.swog.org

Tumor Vaccines
www.tumorvaccines.com

Appendix C: Early Detection Self-Exam Body Map

The four body maps reproduced here, beginning with the front of the body, will help you in prevention and early detection of skin cancer. Make photocopies of the body maps and use them when you examine your skin to mark down the location of each mole. By dating and comparing each month's charts you will easily notice any new moles. For detailed instructions on how to use the body maps, see pages 51–53.

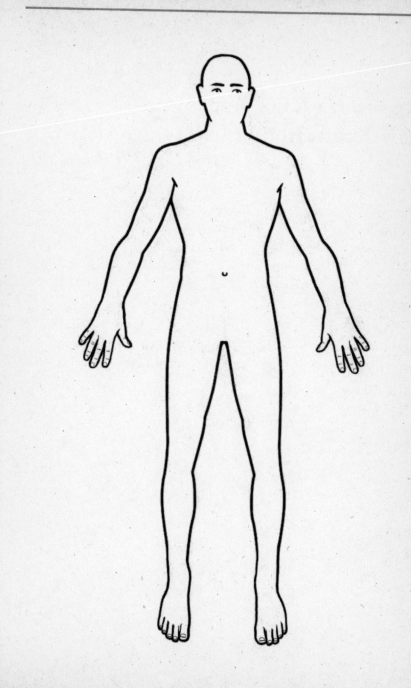

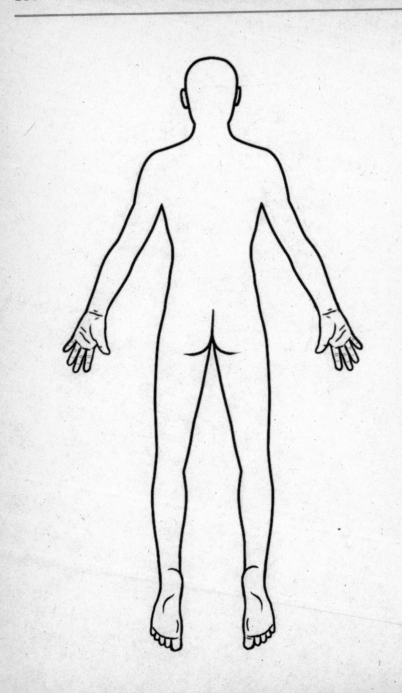

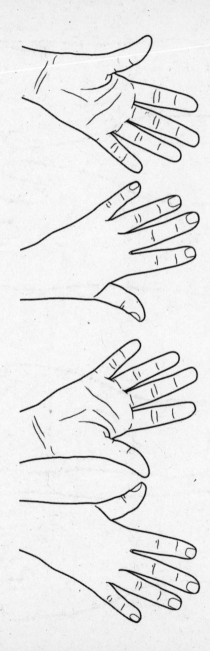

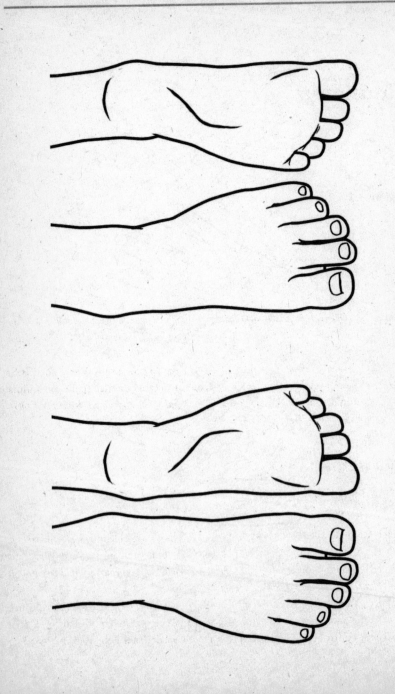

Endnotes

Chapter 1

Cancer Facts and Figures 2004. American Cancer Society, 2004.

Surveillance, Epidemiology, and End Results (SEER) Program, National Cancer Institute, 2004.

Goldsmith, L.A. *Adult And Pediatric Dermatology: A Color Guide to Diagnosis and Treatment*. 1997.

Henneberry J.M., Koch S.E. "Atypical mole syndrome: a brief overview for the primary care physician." *Maryland Medical Journal*. 1997 May–Jun; 46(5):243–6.

Slade, J., Marghoob, A.A., Salopek, T.G., Rigel, D.S., Kopf, A.W., Bart, R.S. "Atypical mole syndrome: risk factor for cutaneous malignant melanoma and implications for management." *Journal of the American Academy of Dermatology*. 1995 Mar; 32(3):479–94.

Chapter 2

Rivers, J.K. "Is there more than one road to melanoma?" *Lancet*. 2004 Feb 28; 363(9410):728–30.

Veierod, M.B., Weiderpass, E., Thorn, M., Hansson, J., Lund, E., Armstrong, B., Adami, H.O. A prospective study of pigmentation, sun exposure, and risk of cutaneous malignant melanoma in women. *Journal of the National Cancer Institute*. 2003 Oct 15; 95(20):1530–8.

Bataille, V., Winnett, A., Sasieni, P., Newton Bishop, J.A., Cuzick, J. Exposure to the sun and sunbeds and the risk of cutaneous melanoma in the UK: a case-control study. *European Journal of Cancer*. 2004 Feb; 40(3):429–35.

Chaudru, V., Chompret, A., Bressac-de Paillerets, B., Spatz, A., Avril, M.F., De-
menais, F. Influence of genes, nevi, and sun sensitivity on melanoma risk in
a family sample unselected by family history and in melanoma-prone families. *Journal of the National Cancer Institute*. 2004 May 19; 96(10):785–95.
Naeyaert, J.M., Brochez, L. Clinical practice. Dysplastic nevi. *New England
Journal of Medicine*. 2003 Dec 4; 349(23):2233–40.

Chapter 3

Oliveria, S.A., Chau, D., Christos, P.J., Charles, C.A., Mushlin, A.I., Halpern,
A.C. Diagnostic accuracy of patients in performing skin self-examination
and the impact of photography. *Archives of Dermatology*. 140(1):57–62,
2004.
Heinzerling, L.M., Dummer, R., Panizzon, R.G., Bloch, P.H., Barbezat, R.,
Burg, G.; Task force 'swiss cancer' of the swiss cancer league. Prevention
campaign against skin cancer. *Dermatology*. 205(3):229–233, 2002.
Dennis, L.K., Beane Freeman, L.E., VanBeek, M.J. Sunscreen use and the risk
for melanoma: a quantitative review. *Annals of Internal Medicine*. 2003 Dec
16; 139(12):966–78.
Beddingfield, F.C. The melanoma epidemic: res ipsa loquitur. *Oncologist*. 2003;
8(5):459–65.
Geller, A.C. Screening for melanoma. *Dermatology Clinics*. 2002 Oct;
20(4):629–40, viii.

Chapter 4

Scolyer, R.A., Thompson, J.F., Stretch, J.R., Sharma, R., McCarthy, S.W. Pathology of melanocytic lesions: new, controversial, and clinically important
issues. *Journal of Surgical Oncology*. 2004 Jul 1; 86(4):200–11.
Barkan, G.A., Rubin, M.A., Michael, C.W. Diagnosis of melanoma aspirates on
ThinPrep: the University of Michigan experience. *Diagnostic Cytopathology*.
2002 May; 26(5):334–9.
Swanson, N.A., Lee, K.K., Gorman, A., Lee, H.N. Biopsy techniques. Diagnosis of melanoma. *Dermatology Clinics*. 2002 Oct; 20(4):677–80.

Pariser, R.J., Divers, A., Nassar, A. The relationship between biopsy technique and uncertainty in the histopathologic diagnosis of melanoma. *Dermatology Online Journal.* 1999 Nov; 5(2):4.

Ruiter, D.J., van Dijk, M.C., Ferrier, C.M. Current diagnostic problems in melanoma pathology. *Seminars in Cutaneous Medicine and Surgery.* 2003 Mar; 22(1):33–41.

Chapter 5

Balch, C.M., Soong, S.J., Atkins, M.B., Buzaid, A.C., Cascinelli, N., Coit, D.G., Fleming, I.D., Gershenwald, J.E., Houghton, A. Jr., Kirkwood, J.M., McMasters, K.M., Mihm, M.F., Morton, D.L., Reintgen, D.S., Ross, M.I., Sober, A., Thompson, J.A., Thompson, J.F. An evidence-based staging system for cutaneous melanoma. *CA Cancer Journal for Clinicians.* 2004 May–Jun; 54(3):131–49.

Schlagenhauff, B., Stroebel, W., Ellwanger, U., Meier, F., Zimmermann, C., Breuninger, H., Rassner, G., Garbe, C. Metastatic melanoma of unknown primary origin shows prognostic similarities to regional metastatic melanoma: recommendations for initial staging examinations. *Cancer.* 1997 Jul 1; 80(1):60–5.

Davids, V., Kidson, S.H., Hanekom, G.S. Melanoma patient staging: histopathological versus molecular evaluation of the sentinel node. *Melanoma Research.* 2003 Jun; 13(3):313–24.

Balch, C.M., Buzaid, A.C., Soong, S.J., Atkins, M.B., Cascinelli, N., Coit, D.G., Fleming, I.D., Gershenwald, J.E., Houghton, A. Jr., Kirkwood, J.M., McMasters, K.M., Mihm, M.F., Morton, D.L., Reintgen, D.S., Ross, M.I., Sober, A., Thompson, J.A., Thompson, J.F. New TNM melanoma staging system: linking biology and natural history to clinical outcomes. *Seminars in Surgical Oncology.* 2003; 21(1):43–52.

Garbe, C., Paul, A., Kohler-Spath, H., Ellwanger, U., Stroebel, W., Schwarz, M., Schlagenhauff, B., Meier, F., Schittek, B., Blaheta, H.J., Blum, A., Rassner, G. Prospective evaluation of a follow-up schedule in cutaneous melanoma patients: recommendations for an effective follow-up strategy. *Journal of Clinical Oncology.* 2003 Feb 1; 21(3):520–9.

Chapter 6

Veronesi, U., Cascinelli, N., Adamus, J., Balch, C., Bandiera, D., Barchuk, A., Bufalino, R., Craig, P., De Marsillac, J., Durand, J.C., et al. Thin stage I primary cutaneous malignant melanoma. Comparison of excision with margins of 1 or 3 cm. *New England Journal of Medicine*. 1988 May 5; 318(18):1159–62.

Thomas, J.M., Newton-Bishop, J., A'Hern, R., Coombes, G., Timmons, M., Evans, J., Cook, M., Theaker, J., Fallowfield, M., O'Neill, T., Ruka, W., Bliss, J.M.; United Kingdom Melanoma Study Group; British Association of Plastic Surgeons; Scottish Cancer Therapy Network. Excision margins in high-risk malignant melanoma. *New England Journal of Medicine*. 2004 Feb 19; 350(8):757–66.

Wagner, J.D., Bergman, D. Primary cutaneous melanoma: surgical management and other treatment options. *Current Treatment Options in Oncology*. 2003 Jun; 4(3):177–85.

Gibson, S.C., Byrne, D.S., McKay, A.J. Ten-year experience of carbon dioxide laser ablation as treatment for cutaneous recurrence of malignant melanoma. *British Journal of Surgery*. 2004 Jul; 91(7):893–5.

Powell, A.M., Russell-Jones, R., Barlow, R.J. Topical imiquimod immunotherapy in the management of lentigo maligna. *Clinical and Experimental Dermatology*. 2004 Jan; 29(1):15–21.

Chapter 7

Cascinelli, N., Morabito, A., Santinami, M., MacKie, R.M., Belli, F. Immediate or delayed dissection of regional nodes in patients with melanoma of the trunk: a randomised trial. WHO Melanoma Programme. *Lancet*. 1998 Mar 14; 351(9105):793–6.

Morton, D.L. Lymphatic mapping and sentinel lymphadenectomy for melanoma: past, present, and future. *Annals of Surgical Oncology*. 2001 Oct; 8(9 Suppl):22S–28S.

Morton, D.L., Chan, A.D. Current status of intraoperative lymphatic mapping and sentinel lymphadenectomy for melanoma: is it standard of care? *Journal of the American College of Surgeons*. 1999 Aug; 189(2):214–23.

Mack, L.A., McKinnon, J.G. Controversies in the management of metastatic melanoma to regional lymphatic basins. *Journal of Surgical Oncology*. 2004 Jul 1; 86(4):189–99.

Kirkwood, J.M., Tarhini, A.A. Adjuvant high-dose interferon-alpha therapy for high-risk melanoma. *Forum* (Genoa). 2003; 13(2):127–43.

Stoutenburg, J., Kaufman, H.L. Adjuvant therapy for melanoma: current status, clinical trials and future directions. *Experimental Reviews in Anticancer Therapy*. 2004 Oct; 4(5):823–35.

Chapter 8

Essner, R. Surgical treatment of malignant melanoma. *Surgical Clinics of North America*. 2003 Feb; 83(1):109–56.

Pavlick, A.C., Adams, S., Fink, M.A., Bailes, A. Novel therapeutic agents under investigation for malignant melanoma. *Expert Opinion in Investigational Drugs*. 2003 Sep; 12(9):1545–58.

Brown, C.K., Kirkwood, J.M. Medical management of melanoma. *Surgical Clinics of North America*. 2003 Apr; 83(2):283–322, viii.

Parmiani, G., Castelli, C., Rivoltini, L., Casati, C., Tully, G.A., Novellino, L., Patuzzo, A., Tosi, D., Anichini, A., Santinami, M. Immunotherapy of melanoma. *Seminars in Cancer Biology*. 2003 Dec; 13(6):391–400.

Atkins, M.B. Interleukin-2: clinical applications. *Seminars in Oncology*. 2002 Jun; 29(3 Suppl 7):12–7.

Chapter 9

Broadbent, A.M., Hruby, G., Tin, M.M., Jackson, M., Firth, I. Survival following whole brain radiation treatment for cerebral metastases: an audit of 474 patients. *Radiotherapy and Oncology*. 2004 Jun; 71(3):259–65.

Robertson, D.M. Changing concepts in the management of choroidal melanoma. *American Journal of Ophthalmology*. 2003 Jul; 136(1):161–70.

Collaborative Ocular Melanoma Study Group. Ten-year follow-up of fellow eyes of patients enrolled in Collaborative Ocular Melanoma Study randomized trials: COMS report no. 22. *Ophthalmology*. 2004 May; 111(5):966–76.

Feldman, E.D., Pingpank, J.F., Alexander, H.R. Jr. Regional treatment options for patients with ocular melanoma metastatic to the liver. *Annals of Surgical Oncology.* 2004 Mar; 11(3):290–7.

Ballo, M.T., Gershenwald, J.E., Zagars, G.K., Lee, J.E., Mansfield, P.F., Strom, E.A., Bedikian, A.Y., Kim, K.B., Papadopoulos, N.E., Prieto, V.G., Ross, M.I. Sphincter-sparing local excision and adjuvant radiation for anal-rectal melanoma. *Journal of Clinical Oncology.* 2002 Dec 1; 20(23):4555–8.

Chapter 10

Poo-Hwu, W.J., Ariyan, S., Lamb, L., Papac, R., Zelterman, D., Hu, G.L., Brown, J., Fischer, D., Bolognia, J., Buzaid, A.C. Follow-up recommendations for patients with American Joint Committee on Cancer Stages I-III malignant melanoma. *Cancer.* 1999 Dec 1; 86(11):2252–8.

Christianson, D.F., Anderson, C.M. Close monitoring and lifetime follow-up is optimal for patients with a history of melanoma. *Seminars in Oncology.* 2003 Jun; 30(3):369–74.

Garbe, C. A rational approach to the follow-up of melanoma patients. Recent Results. *Cancer Research.* 2002; 160:205–15.

Diener-West, M., Reynolds, S.M., Agugliaro, D.J., Caldwell, R., Cumming, K., Earle, J.D., Green, D.L., Hawkins, B.S., Hayman, J., Jaiyesimi, I., Kirkwood, J.M., Koh, W.J., Robertson, D.M., Shaw, J.M., Thoma, J.; Collaborative Ocular Melanoma Study Group Report 23. Screening for metastasis from choroidal melanoma: the Collaborative Ocular Melanoma Study Group Report 23. *Journal of Clinical Oncology.* 2004 Jun 15; 22(12):2438–44.

Finkelstein, S.E., Carrasquillo, J.A., Hoffman, J.M., Galen, B., Choyke, P., White, D.E., Rosenberg, S.A., Sherry, R.M. A Prospective Analysis of Positron Emission Tomography and Conventional Imaging for Detection of Stage IV Metastatic Melanoma in Patients Undergoing Metastasectomy. *Annals of Surgical Oncology.* 2004 Jul 12: 731–8.

Chapter 11

Slavin, K.V., Tesoro, E.P., Mucksavage, J.J. The treatment of cancer pain. *Drugs Today* (Barcelona). 2004 Mar; 40(3):235–45.

Oldham, L., Kristjanson, L.J. Development of a pain management programme for family carers of advanced cancer patients. *International Journal of Palliative Nursing*. 2004 Feb; 10(2):91–9.

Hall, E.J., Sykes, N.P. Analgesia for patients with advanced disease: I. *Postgraduate Medical Journal*. 2004 Mar; 80(941):148–54.

Ferrell, B.R., Rivera, L.M. Cancer pain education for patients. *Seminars in Oncology Nursing*. 1997 Feb; 13(1):42–8.

Caraceni, A., Martini, C., Zecca, E., Portenoy, R.K., Ashby, M.A., Hawson, G., Jackson, K.A., Lickiss, N., Muirden, N., Pisasale, M., Moulin, D., Schulz, V.N., Rico Pazo, M.A., Serrano, J.A., Andersen, H., Henriksen, H.T., Mejholm, I., Sjogren, P., Heiskanen, T., Kalso, E., Pere, P., Poyhia, R., Vuorinen, E., Tigerstedt, I., Ruismaki, P., Bertolino, M., Larue, F., Ranchere, J.Y., Hege-Scheuing, G., Bowdler, I., Helbing, F., Kostner, E., Radbruch, L., Kastrinaki, K., Shah, S., Vijayaram, S., Sharma, K.S., Devi, P.S., Jain, P.N., Ramamani, P.V., Beny, A., Brunelli, C., Maltoni, M., Mercadante, S., Plancarte, R., Schug, S., Engstrand, P., Ovalle, A.F., Wang, X., Alves, M.F., Abrunhosa, M.R., Sun, W.Z., Zhang, L., Gazizov, A., Vaisman, M., Rudoy, S., Gomez Sancho, M., Vila, P., Trelis, J., Chaudakshetrin, P., Koh, M.L., Van Dongen, R.T., Vielvoye-Kerkmeer, A., Boswell, M.V., Elliott, T., Hargus, E., Lutz, L.; Working Group of an IASP Task Force on Cancer Pain. Breakthrough pain characteristics and syndromes in patients with cancer pain. An international survey. *Palliative Medicine*. 2004 Apr; 18(3):177–83.

Chapter 12

Bukowski, R.M., Tendler, C., Cutler, D., Rose, E., Laughlin, M.M., Statkevich, P. Treating cancer with PEG Intron: pharmacokinetic profile and dosing guidelines for an improved interferon-alpha-2b formulation. *Cancer*. 2002 Jul 15; 95(2):389–96.

Cassell, D.J., Choudhri, S., Humphrey, R., Martell, R.E., Reynolds, T., Shanafelt, A.B. Therapeutic enhancement of IL-2 through molecular design. *Current Pharmaceutical Design*. 2002; 8(24):2171–83.

Spitler, L.E., Grossbard, M.L., Ernstoff, M.S., Silver, G., Jacobs, M., Hayes,

F.A., Soong, S.J. Adjuvant therapy of stage III and IV malignant melanoma using granulocyte-macrophage colony-stimulating factor. *Journal of Clinical Oncology.* 2000 Apr; 18(8):1614–21.

Atkins, M.B., Robertson, M.J., Gordon, M., Lotze, M.T., DeCoste, M., DuBois, J.S., Ritz, J., Sandler, A.B., Edington, H.D., Garzone, P.D., Mier, J.W., Canning, C.M., Battiato, L., Tahara, H., Sherman, M.L. Phase I evaluation of intravenous recombinant human interleukin 12 in patients with advanced malignancies. *Clinical Cancer Research.* 1997 Mar; 3(3):409–17.

Finkelstein, S.E., Heimann, D.M., Klebanoff, C.A., Antony, P.A., Gattinoni, L., Hinrichs, C.S., Hwang, L.N., Palmer, D.C., Spiess, P.J., Surman, D.R., Wrzesiniski, C., Yu, Z., Rosenberg, S.A., Restifo, N.P. Bedside to bench and back again: how animal models are guiding the development of new immunotherapies for cancer. *Journal of Leukocyte Biology.* 2004 May 20 [Epub ahead of print].

Chapter 13

Komenaka, I., Hoerig, H., Kaufman, H.L. Immunotherapy for melanoma. *Clinics in Dermatology.* 2004; 22(3):251–65.

Pardoll, D.M. Spinning molecular immunology into successful immunotherapy. *Nature Reviews Immunology.* 2002 Apr; 2(4):227–38.

Gilboa, E. The promise of cancer vaccines. *Nature Reviews Cancer.* 2004 May; 4(5):401–11.

Dunn, G.P., Old, L.J., Schreiber, R.D. The three Es of cancer immunoediting. *Annual Reviews in Immunology.* 2004; 22:329–60.

Horig, H., Kaufman, H.L. Local delivery of poxvirus vaccines for melanoma. *Seminars in Cancer Biology.* 2003 Dec; 13(6):417–22.

Chapter 14

Ruf, P., Jager, M., Ellwart, J., Wosch, S., Kusterer, E., Lindhofer, H. Two new trifunctional antibodies for the therapy of human malignant melanoma. *International Journal of Cancer.* 2004 Feb 20; 108(5):725–32.

Hwu, W.J., Krown, S.E., Menell, J.H., Panageas, K.S., Merrell, J., Lamb, L.A., Williams, L.J., Quinn, C.J., Foster, T., Chapman, P.B., Livingston, P.O., Wolchok, J.D., Houghton, A.N. Phase II study of temozolomide plus thalidomide for the treatment of metastatic melanoma. *Journal of Clinical Oncology.* 2003 Sep 1; 21(17):3351–6.

Fiorentini, G., Rossi, S., Lanzanova, G., Bernardeschi, P., Dentico, P., De Giorgi, U. Potential use of imatinib mesylate in ocular melanoma and liposarcoma expressing immunohistochemical c-KIT (CD117). *Annals of Oncology.* 2003 May; 14(5):805.

Karasarides, M., Chiloeches, A., Hayward, R., Niculescu-Duvaz, D., Scanlon, I., Friedlos, F., Ogilvie, L., Hedley, D., Martin, J., Marshall, C.J., Springer, C.J., Marais, R. B-RAF is a therapeutic target in melanoma. *Oncogene.* 2004 Jun 21 [Epub ahead of print].

Edelstein, M.L., Abedi, M.R., Wixon, J., Edelstein, R.M. Gene therapy clinical trials worldwide 1989–2004—an overview. *Journal of Gene Medicine.* 2004 Jun; 6(6):597–602.

Chapter 15

Carlson, R.V., Boyd, K.M., Webb, D.J. The revision of the Declaration of Helsinki: past, present and future. *British Journal of Clinical Pharmacology.* 2004 Jun; 57(6):695–713.

Kapp, M.B. Regulating hematology/oncology research involving human participants. *Hematology and Oncology Clinics of North America.* 2002 Dec; 16(6):1449–61.

World Health Organization. International Ethical Guidelines for Biomedical Research Involving Human Subjects. Available from the *Council for International Organizations of Medical Sciences (CIOMS).* E-mail: cioms@who.int.

U.S. Food and Drug Administration. Protection of human subjects; informed consent; proposed rule. *Federal Register.* 1995 Sep 21; 60(183):49086–103.

The National Commission for the Protection of Human Subjects of Biomedical and Behavioral Research. The Belmont Report: Ethical Principles and Guidelines for the Protection of Human Subjects of Research. Available at www.brown.edu/Administration/Research_Administration/belmont/belmont.html.

Glossary

ACRAL LENTIGINOUS MELANOMA: A type of melanoma typically found on the palms of the hands or soles of the feet that appears as an irregular brown patch and has a somewhat worse prognosis than other types of melanoma.

ACTINIC KERATOSES: A precancerous condition of flat, pink, scaly spots that grow on sun-damaged skin of older, fair-skinned people.

ACUTE PAIN: Short-lasting often severe pain; usually manifests in ways that can be easily described and observed. Sometimes causes sweating or increased heart rate.

ADENO-ASSOCIATED VIRUS: A small, stable virus not known to cause disease in humans and used for gene therapy. The naturally occurring form of the virus has only two genes, which are removed and replaced by therapeutic genes for gene therapy studies.

ADENOVIRUS: A virus that can cause respiratory and eye infections. It is being studied as a way to deliver therapeutic genes as part of gene therapy, for melanoma and other diseases.

ADJUVANT THERAPY: Any type of therapy used after primary cancer treatment to decrease the chance of cancer recurrence.

ADOPTIVE TRANSFER THERAPY: Form of passive immunization where previously sensitized immunologic agents (such as T cells or antibodies) are transferred to a patient.

ADVERSE EVENT: A term used for a side effect (expected or unexpected) that occurs while a patient is on a clinical trial.

ALDARA CREAM: A substance used for treating common skin warts and possibly for basal cell carcinoma. Although still experimental, Aldara cream activates the local immune response and may prove useful for the treatment of other types of skin cancer.

ALLOGENEIC VACCINES: Vaccines made from tumor cells taken from individuals other than the patient.

AMELANOTIC MELANOMA: A form of melanoma in which the malignant cells (melanocytes) do not make the pigment melanin. Amelanotic melanomas may be pink, red, or have light brown, tan, or gray at the edges and are usually detectable only on close examination of the skin.

ANAL MELANOMA: An aggressive form of melanoma that occurs around the anus and is easily confused with benign hemorrhoids.

ANEMIA: A deficiency in the oxygen-carrying component of the blood due to a loss of hemoglobin or red blood cells. Anemia can be caused by melanoma and is a common side effect of chemotherapy.

ANGIOGENESIS: The process by which new blood vessels are produced. This process may play a role in promoting the growth of melanomas and has been a target for new treatment strategies.

ANTI-ANGIOGENESIS: The prevention of angiogenesis (new blood vessel formation), a goal for anti-cancer strategies where tumors are killed by cutting off their blood supply.

ANTIBODIES: A protein substance produced in the blood or tissues in response to a specific antigen, such as a bacterium or a toxin, which destroys bacteria and neutralizes organic poisons. Antibodies may be formed naturally against proteins found on melanoma cells in some patients or may be made artificially in the laboratory for cancer therapy.

ANTIBODY-DEPENDENT CELL CYTOTOXICITY: A process whereby antibodies cause the death of specific cells; the antibody attaches to a single protein and signals other cells in the immune system to destroy the targeted cell. This is one mechanism by which the immune system may be able to destroy melanoma cells.

ANTIGEN: A substance recognized as foreign by the immune system; may trigger an immune response.

ATYPICAL FIBROXANTHOMA: A tumor that occurs primarily in older individuals after the skin of the head and neck has been damaged significantly by sun exposure and/or radiation therapy. These lesions may arise rapidly (over just a few weeks or months) in areas where other skin cancers have been found and treated.

ATYPICAL NEVUS: A mole whose appearance differs from that of common moles in one or more ways. Atypical moles may be larger than ordinary moles, and may have irregular or indistinct borders, with variations of color within the mole. They usually are flat, but parts may be raised above the skin surface. Also known as a dysplastic nevus, these lesions are thought to be the precursor of a true melanoma. Atypical nevi should be removed.

AUTOIMMUNITY: A misdirected immune response that occurs when the immune system goes awry and attacks the body itself.

AUTOLOGOUS VACCINES: Vaccines made from molecules or cells taken from a patient's own body.

AVASTIN® (BEVACIZUMAB): A monoclonal antibody that targets one of the angiogenesis factors. Avastin was approved for the treatment of colon cancer when given in combination with chemotherapy and is being evaluated in other cancers.

AXILLARY LYMPH NODE DISSECTION: A surgical procedure involving the removal of the lymph nodes under the armpit (axillary nodes).

BACILLUS CALMETTE GUERIN (BCG): A bacterium that is related to the tuberculosis bacterium and is used to prevent tuberculosis and as a general immunologic booster in many cancer vaccines.

BASAL CELL CARCINOMA: A type of skin cancer that arises from the basal cells, usually found on sun exposed parts of the body and readily cured by surgical excision in most cases.

BASAL CELLS: Round cells found in the innermost layer of the epidermis.

B CELLS: A major class of lymphocytes, these cells produce and secrete antibodies.

BIOCHEMOTHERAPY: The combination of chemotherapy and immunotherapy being investigated as a treatment approach for melanoma.

BIOPSY: The removal and examination of a sample of tissue from a living body for diagnostic purposes.

BIOSTATISTICS: The analysis of biological or medical data.

BIOTHERAPY: Treatment of disease with biological agents, such as cytokines and vaccines.

BISPHOSPHONATES: A class of drugs developed as calcium-lowering agents, which also control cancer related bone pain.

BRAF GENE: A gene that encodes a type of kinase which functions to control cell functions. This gene is abnormal or mutated in many melanoma cells.

Inhibition of BRAF activity may be a useful new therapeutic strategy for metastatic melanoma.

BREAKTHROUGH PAIN: A brief flare-up of chronic pain that occurs even while the patient is regularly taking pain medication.

CALCITONIN: A peptide hormone, produced by the thyroid gland in humans, which lowers plasma calcium and phosphate levels without augmenting calcium secretion. May help control difficult bone pain.

CANCER: A condition whereby normal cells of the body divide without control. In benign cancers the cells enlarge and can disrupt the normal surrounding body tissues. In malignant cancers, the cells can travel throughout the body and replace normal body tissues in many other locations. See also lesions, nodules, and tumor.

CANCER CELLS: Cells of the body that undergo uncontrolled growth and division. These cells can invade nearby tissues and can spread through the bloodstream and lymphatic system to various parts of the body.

CARMUSTINE (BCNU): A type of chemotherapy used to treat melanoma.

CAT (OR CT) SCAN (COMPUTERIZED AXIAL TOMOGRAPHY SCAN): An X-ray test that is used in diagnostic studies of internal body structures. Computer analysis is used to construct a three-dimensional image of a body structure or tissue. Useful for evaluating the chest, abdomen, and pelvis in melanoma patients.

CHEMOKINE: Small molecule that attracts and activates leukocytes and other cells of the immune system.

CHEMOTHERAPY: The treatment of cancer using specific chemical agents or drugs that destroys actively dividing cells, including cancer cells, normal blood cells, hair follicles, and cells of the gastrointestinal tract.

CHRONIC PAIN: Pain lasting more than three months. The body may become accustomed to such pain.

CILIARY BODY: A thickened portion of the vascular tunic of the eye between the choroid and the iris.

CISPLATIN (DDP): A type of chemotherapy used to treat melanoma.

CLINICAL TRIAL: An experimental study that tests the effects of a new vaccine or drug in patients with cancer.

COLONY-STIMULATING FACTORS: Substances that stimulate the production of new blood cells. Colony-stimulating factors include granulocyte colony-stimulating factor (also called G-CSF and filgrastim), granulocyte-macrophage colony-stimulating factors (also called GM-CSF and sargramostim), erythropoietin, and promegapoietin.

COMPLETE RESPONSE: Complete disappearance of all measurable cancer for at least four weeks.

COMPREHENSIVE CANCER CENTER: Specialized centers providing complete care for patients with cancer. Also offers basic, clinical, and population-based cancer research programs.

CONJUNCTIVA: The mucous membrane lining the inner eyelid and the exposed surface of the eyeball.

CONTROL GROUP: A group of patients used as a standard for comparison in an experimental clinical trial.

CO-STIMULATORY MOLECULE: A molecule that provides additional signals for lymphocyte activation beyond those provided through the antigen receptor.

CUTANEOUS MELANOMA: Melanoma that starts in the skin.

CYCLOPHOSPHAMIDE: A type of chemotherapy.

CYTOKINES: Small proteins produced naturally in the body that stimulate the activity of immune cells. Some cytokines are used for the treatment of melanoma, such as interferon-alpha and interleukin-2.

DACARBAZINE (OR DTIC): A type of chemotherapy used to treat melanoma.

DATA SAFETY MONITORING BOARD: An independent committee that monitors adverse events related to clinical protocols and makes recommendations for changes in a clinical trial.

DEEP INGUINAL LYMPH NODE DISSECTION: A surgical procedure that removes lymph nodes in the groin and deeper parts of the pelvis.

DENDRITIC CELLS: Antigen-presenting cells characterized by their fingerlike or dendrite extensions. These cells start an immune response by activating T cells and B cells.

DENDRITIC CELL VACCINES: Vaccines that use dendritic cells to carry and present tumor antigens to the immune system, activating an immune response against the cancer.

DERMATOPATHOLOGIST: A pathologist with additional training and certification in diseases of the skin; often makes the diagnosis of melanoma from skin biopsies.

DERMIS: The deeper layer of the skin located below the epidermis.

DESMOPLASTIC MELANOMA: A rare form of aggressive malignant melanoma marked by non-pigmented lesions on sun-exposed body parts, most commonly on the head and neck.

DNA (DEOXYRIBONUCLEIC ACID): Often called "the blueprint of life," this nucleic acid carries the cell's genetic information (genes) and hereditary characteristics.

DNA VACCINE: A vaccine in which DNA containing an antigen or immune stimulating gene is injected and expressed in host cells; the expressed antigen stimulates an immune response.

DOCETAXEL (TAXOTERE): A type of chemotherapy used to treat melanoma.

DYSPLASTIC NEVUS: See *Atypical nevus.*

DYSPLASTIC NEVUS SYNDROME: A genetic condition characterized by the appearance of many atypical nevi of the skin. Patients with dyspastic nevus syndrome have an increased risk of melanoma, which often occurs at a younger age. Patients should be followed very closely by a trained dermatologist who can biopsy any changing moles.

EKG—ELECTROCARDIOGRAM: An instrument used in the detection and diagnosis of heart abnormalities that generates a record of the electrical currents of the heart.

ENDOTHELIAL CELLS: The main type of cell found on the inside lining of blood vessels, lymph vessels, and the heart.

ENUCLEATE: To completely remove something, such as an eye.

ENZYME: A protein that speeds up chemical reactions in the body.

EPHELIDES: Freckles; may be a risk factor for skin cancer, including melanoma.

EPIDERMIS: The nonvascular outer layer of the skin, protecting the dermis.

ERBITUX® (CETUXIMAB): A type of monoclonal antibody that targets a growth receptor on cancer cells and is being studied as an anticancer drug.

EXCISION: Surgical removal by cutting, as of a tumor or a portion of a structure or organ.

EXTERNAL BEAM RADIATION THERAPY: Radiation therapy administered from an energy source outside the body and directed to a target inside the body.

FAMILIAL MELANOMA SYNDROME: An inherited syndrome where family members develop melanoma. The disease is usually diagnosed at an early age and patients have multiple primary sites. The diagnosis of this syndrome requires at least two first-degree relatives to have melanoma.

FENTANYL: A strong pain medication used during an operation and for cancer pain control.

FINE NEEDLE ASPIRATION (FNA): A "through-the-skin" procedure that takes fluid from a cyst or removes clusters of cells from a solid mass. This minor procedure can be done in the office and usually enough tissue is removed for microscopic analysis to make an accurate diagnosis of melanoma.

FOTEMUSTINE: A type of chemotherapy used to treat melanoma.

GAMMA KNIFE RADIOSURGERY: An advanced form of stereotactic or focused radiosurgery for brain tumors or melanoma in the brain. The "knife" is formed by 201 intersecting beams of gamma radiation that deliver a concentrated dose to a precise area of the brain.

GANCICLOVIR: An antiviral drug used to prevent or treat viral infections that may occur when the body's immune system is suppressed. This drug has also been used in experimental gene therapy clinical trials.

GASTROINTESTINAL STROMAL TUMOR (GIST): A rare type of tumor that usually begins in cells in the wall of the gastrointestinal tract.

GENE THERAPY: The introduction of new genetic material to cells in the body. Gene therapy is a method for replacing damaged genes in cancer cells with healthy ones, or to make cancer cells more sensitive to the effects of the immune system, immunotherapy, or chemotherapy.

GLEEVEC® (IMATINIB MESYLATE): A new type of drug that blocks the kinase pathway in some cancer cells, preventing cell growth and division. Gleevec has been approved for treatment of malignant gastrointestinal stromal tumor (GIST) and chronic myeloid leukemia.

GM-CSF (GRANULOCYTE MACROPHAGE COLONY-STIMULATING FACTOR): A naturally produced immune system protein (or cytokine) that stimulates the production of white blood cells. Currently being investigated as a treatment for melanoma.

GP100: A common melanoma antigen that can be found on melanoma cells from a biopsy specimen.

GROWTH FACTORS: Substances made by the body that regulate cell division and cell survival. Some growth factors are also produced in the laboratory and used in biological therapy.

HEAT SHOCK PROTEINS (HSPS): A family of proteins found in all cells that are expressed in response to cold, heat, and other environmental stresses. HSPs may help start an immune response and HSPs from melanoma cells have been tested as vaccines.

HERCEPTIN® (TRASTUZUMAB): A monoclonal antibody that targets a protein called Her-2/neu, found in some cases of breast and other types of cancer. Herceptin has been useful in the treatment of breast cancer when given in combination with chemotherapy.

HLA TYPING: A blood test that determines which human leukocyte antigens (HLA) are present on the cells of a patient. This information is required to determine if certain peptide vaccines will be able to bind to the patient's HLA complex and trigger an immune response.

HUMAN LEUKOCYTE ANTIGEN (HLA): The major, genetically-determined antigen compatibility complex in humans; HLA allows immune cells to distinguish cells from the same body ("self") from those cells not belonging to the body ("non-self"), such as infections, transplants, and possibly cancer cells.

HUMAN PAPILLOMA VIRUS: A family of over one hundred viruses including those that cause warts and are transmitted by contact. Vaccines for certain papilloma viruses, such as HPV-16 and HPV-18, are being studied in clinical trials for the prevention of cervical cancer.

HYPERTHERMIA: A process of heating the body used to enhance a drug's potency.

IMMUNE SYSTEM: The system of organs, tissues, and cells that identifies foreign bodies, such as infected cells and cancer cells, and neutralizes potentially dangerous organisms, cells, and substances.

IMMUNOLOGY: The branch of biomedicine concerned with the structure and function of the immune system.

IMMUNOTHERAPY: The use of natural or manufactured substances to help the body's immune system fight disease more effectively.

INFORMED CONSENT: A process in which you learn the facts about a clinical trial, including the reasons for the study, the procedures involved, the risks and benefits, the alternative treatments available, and the costs, before deciding whether to participate.

INGUINAL LYMPH NODE DISSECTION: A surgical procedure in which the groin lymph nodes are removed and examined to see whether they contain cancer.

IN SITU: In the original position; refers to melanoma that has not moved below the epidermis. These lesions are curable with surgical removal.

INSTITUTIONAL REVIEW BOARD (IRB): A local institutional committee that evaluates all clinical trials to ensure protection of human subjects.

INTERFERON: Natural proteins produced by normal cells in response to viral infections and disease, including cancer. Interferons affect immune responses and boost resistance to viral infection. Interferon therapies have been shown to help the body's immune system fight disease more effectively and may inhibit the growth of blood vessels that feed cancer cells.

INTERFERON ALPHA: One of three major species of interferon produced by the body. It has been found most useful in treating forms of cancer, including Stage III melanoma, leukemia, and possibly kidney cancer.

INTERLEUKINS: A family of substances produced naturally in the body in response to infections; they help the immune system produce more infection- and cancer-fighting cells.

INTERLEUKIN-2 (IL-2): A naturally produced protein of the immune system that stimulates the growth of specific types of white blood cells. It is an FDA-approved immunotherapy for Stage IV melanoma and kidney cancer.

INTERLEUKIN-12 (IL-12): A cytokine very similar to IL-2 that acts as a growth factor for T cells and natural killer (NK) cells. IL-12 also causes the cells to produce interferon-gamma, another cytokine important for fighting cancer.

INTERLEUKIN-15 (IL-15): A new cytokine that has similar activity to IL-2. IL-15 stimulates the growth of T cells, B cells, and NK cells.

INTERLEUKIN-18 (IL-18): A cytokine similar to IL-12 that helps stimulate T cells. IL-18 has shown anti-tumor activity in animal models.

INTERLEUKIN-21 (IL-21): An IL-2–related cytokine that stimulates T and NK cell responses with anti-tumor activity in animal models.

INTERLEUKIN-23 (IL-23): An IL-12–related cytokine thast helps promote immune responses and has shown activity against melanoma in animal studies.

INTERNAL RADIATION THERAPY: The delivery of radioactive material to a location very close to the tumor from a source placed inside the body. Methods of delivery include injection, ingestion, or implantation. Also known as brachytherapy.

INTERVENTIONAL RADIOLOGY: A subspecialty within the field of radiology that uses various radiology techniques (such as X-ray, CT scans, MRI scans, and ultrasounds) to place wires, tubes, or other instruments inside a patient to diagnose or treat an array of conditions.

IN-TRANSIT MELANOMA: A condition where melanoma nodules can be felt along the path of normal lymphatic drainage, usually occurring between a known skin melanoma site and the closest lymph node basin.

INTRAVENEOUS CATHETER: A hollow, flexible tube inserted into a vein so fluids and/or medicines can be given.

INVESTIGATOR-INITIATED STUDY: A study by an individual or group of research investigators, as opposed to a study sponsored by a pharmaceutical or biotechnology company.

IRIS: The round, pigmented eye membrane surrounding the pupil responsible for the color of the eyes.

ISOLATED LIMB PERFUSION: A technique that delivers anticancer drugs directly to an arm or leg through an isolated circulatory circuit. This may be useful for in-transit melanoma of the arms and legs.

KILLER CELL: A large differentiated T cell that attacks and kills target cells bearing specific antigens, such as virus infected or cancer cells.

LACTATE DEHYDROGENASE (LDH): An enzyme found in the blood and many body tissues such as the liver, kidney, brain, and lungs. LDH levels are determined by a simple blood test and elevated levels of LDH may indicate the presence of advanced melanoma.

LASER PHOTOCOAGULATION: A procedure that uses laser to coagulate tissue with intense light energy, destroying abnormal tissues or forming adhesive scars, especially useful in ophthalmology.

LASER THERAPY: The use of an intensely powerful beam of light to kill cancer cells.

LENTIGO: A flat, brown spot associated with aging or sun-damaged skin; also known as sunspots, age spots, or liver spots.

LENTIGO MALIGNA MELANOMA: Melanoma arising from a lentigo rather than a mole, and representing about 5 percent of all melanomas. It occurs most often in older women, usually on the face and other chronically sun-exposed areas. The melanomas are generally large, flat, tan-colored lesions and have a better prognosis than most other forms of melanoma.

LESION: A general term for an abnormal area of the body, including a cancer, nodule, mass, tumor, or melanoma.

LIDOCAINE: A synthetic drug used as a local anesthetic and anti-arrhythmic agent.

LIPOMA: A benign fatty tumor, which commonly occurs just under the skin and can be felt.

LOCAL ABLATION THERAPY: A variety of techniques in which small melanoma nodules are destroyed. A carbon dioxide laser has been very successful in removing small lesions with few recurrences. More experimental methods include photodynamic therapy and local bleomycin injection with electrical impulses applied to the lesions.

LOCAL RESECTION: Removal of a tumor and a small portion of the surrounding tissue by a surgical procedure.

LOMUSTINE (CCNU): A type of chemotherapy used to treat melanoma.

LYMPHATIC MAPPING: A procedure in which a tiny amount of radioactive tracer or colored dye is injected into the skin to map the way lymph drains from a melanoma to its closest lymph nodes. When a radioactive tracer is used a scan of the tracer can be obtained to form a picture of where the lymph node is found; this procedure is also known as lymphoscintigraphy.

LYMPH NODES: Pea-size organs distributed throughout the body that filter lymph, trap foreign bodies (including cancer cells), and fight infection and disease. Since lymph nodes receive drainage from melanoma cells, they are often the first site for spread or metastasis. The largest collections of lymph nodes are in the neck, under the armpits, and in the groin.

LYMPHOCELE: A pocket of lymph accumulation at the site of lymph node removal.

LYMPHOCYTES: A type of the white blood cell formed in lymphoid tissue (includes the lymph nodes, spleen, thymus, and tonsils) that circulates through the body to fight disease. The two major types of lymphocytes are B cells that produce antibodies and T cells that directly kill infected and cancerous cells.

LYMPHOMA: Cancer that arises in cells of the lymphatic system.

MACROPHAGE: A type of white blood cell that kills microorganisms, removes dead cells, and stimulates other immune system cells.

MAGE-3: A melanoma antigen.

MAGNETIC RESONANCE IMAGING (MRI): A diagnostic technique in which magnetic fields create detailed, cross-sectional images of the body. An MRI is commonly used to detect melanoma in the brain or other locations.

MAJOR HISTOCOMPATIBILITY COMPLEX (MHC): A set of molecular complexes that allows immune cells to recognize cells from the same body ("self") from those cells not belonging to the body ("non-self"), such as infections, transplants, and possible cancer cells. In humans the MHC are called human leukocyte antigens (HLA).

MALIGNANT: Cancerous; describing cells that invade and destroy nearby tissue and spread to other parts of the body.

MART-1: A common melanoma antigen that can be found on melanoma cells from a biopsy specimen.

MELANIN: A pigment produced by melanocytes that gives color to the skin, hair, and parts of the eye, providing protection against the damaging effects of ultraviolet radiation.

MELANOCYTES: Melanin-producing cells located in the deep layers of the epidermis.

MELANOMA: A type of skin cancer arising from melanocytes in the skin, mucous membranes, or eye with potential for spreading to almost any organ in the body.

MELANOMA-ASSOCIATED GENE 1 (MAGE-1): A common melanoma antigen.

MELPHALAN: A type of chemotherapy agent commonly used in isolated limb perfusions for melanoma.

MEMORY CELLS: A subset of T or B cells that remain in the body after being exposed to a particular antigen. Memory cells can mount an immediate immune attack if the body is invaded by the same organism or cancer cell.

MERKEL CELL CARCINOMA: An infrequent but highly malignant type of skin cancer. Characteristically starts in a sun-exposed area as a firm, painless, shiny lump that can be red, pink, or blue and vary in size from less than a quarter of an inch to more than two inches in diameter. Treatment is surgical removal and radiation therapy in most cases.

METASTASIS (METASTATIC CANCER): A process where malignant cancer spreads from one area of the body to another. The treatment is based on the site of the original cancer, not on the organ it spreads to. For example, melanoma that spreads to the lungs is treated as melanoma, not lung cancer.

METHADONE: A synthetic narcotic drug used to alleviate pain from cancer and also used as a substitute narcotic in the treatment of heroin addiction.

MICROCYSTIC ADNEXAL CARCINOMA: A rare, malignant appendage tumor commonly classified as a low-grade sweat gland cancer. It shows aggressive local invasion but has little metastatic potential.

MODIFIED RADICAL NECK DISSECTION: A surgical procedure for removing lymph nodes from the neck.

MOHS MICROGRAPHIC SURGERY: A technique involving the sequential removal of a skin cancer with immediate microscopic examination to determine if cancer cells are present. The dissection continues as long as cancer is still present in the specimen. This allows removal of minimum tissue but assures that all cancer is removed. At present, the Mohs technique is especially useful for basal cell carcinoma but is not recommended for melanoma since it can miss areas of melanoma.

MOLE: A pigmented skin growth most commonly formed by a cluster of melanocytes and surrounding supportive tissue. Moles usually appear as tan, brown, or flesh-colored spots on the skin; also called nevi.

MONOCLONAL ANTIBODY: A type of highly specific antibody that targets a single antigen. Monoclonal antibodies are widely used in biomedical research and as therapeutic agents in adoptive immunotherapy.

MORPHINE: A bitter crystalline alkaloid extracted from opium, the soluble salts of which are used in medicine as an analgesic, a light anesthetic, or a sedative.

MUCOSAL MELANOMA: An uncommon type of melanoma that occurs in mucosal regions of the mouth, nose, and genitals.

MULTIPLE MYELOMA: A type of cancer that arises from the antibody producing cells known as plasma cells.

MUTATION: A permanent change in the genetic, inherited structural DNA of a cell that may cause it to become cancerous.

NAPROXEN: A drug used to reduce inflammation and pain, especially in the treatment of arthritis or cancer.

NATURAL KILLER (NK) CELLS: A type of lymphocyte, or white blood cell, that attacks virus infected cells and possibly cancer cells. There is less known about the role of NK cells in cancer but there is strong evidence that these cells play a part in killing cancer cells.

NERVE BLOCK: Interruption of the passages of impulses through a nerve cell by the injection of alcohol or an anesthetic drug; often effective for the treatment of neuropathic pain.

NEUROPATHIC PAIN: Pain caused by injuring a nerve as a result of a cancer compressing the nerve. Neuropathic pain may also result from chemical damage to the nervous system caused by cancer treatment (chemotherapy, radiation, surgery). This type of pain is severe and usually described as burning or tingling.

NEUROPATHY: A disease or an abnormality of the nervous system, especially one affecting the nerves outside of the brain or spinal cord. This is a common side effect of some types of chemotherapy and often results in numbness or tingling over the fingers and toes.

NEVUS: The medical term for a mole.

NODULAR MELANOMA: Type of melanoma that usually appears as a blue-black, dome-shaped nodule and has an intermediate prognosis.

NODULE: A small lump, mass of tissue, or aggregation of cells. See also *cancer*, *lesion*, and *tumor*.

NON-PIGMENTED SKIN LESIONS: Lesions on the skin that contain very little coloring. Non-pigmented lesions include warts, skin tags, and occasionally melanomas. However, melanoma is more commonly found in pigmented skin lesions.

NUCLEAR MEDICINE: The branch of medicine that deals with the use of radionuclides in the diagnosis and treatment of disease.

NY-ESO-1: A melanoma antigen.

OCULAR MELANOMA: A malignant melanoma arising from a structure within the eye.

ONCOGENE: An abnormal gene that allows uncontrolled growth and division of a particular cell leading to cancer. The genetic alterations can be inherited or caused by environmental exposure to carcinogens.

OPHTHALMOSCOPE: An instrument for examining the interior structures of the eye, especially the retina. It consists of a mirror that reflects light into the eye and a central hole through which the eye is examined.

OXYCODONE: A narcotic alkaloid related to codeine, used as an analgesic and a sedative for control of cancer pain.

PACLITAXEL (TAXOL): A type of chemotherapy used to treat melanoma.

PALLIATIVE TREATMENT: Treatment that alleviates symptoms without curing the disease.

PARTIAL RESPONSE: A measurement of how well cancer has responded to a particular treatment or intervention. A partial response implies that there is greater than 50 percent decrease in the amount of cancer and no evidence of new cancer after treatment.

PEPTIDES: A small fragment of a protein composed of several amino acids, the building blocks of proteins. Most T cells recognize antigens only after being processed into peptides and binding to HLA complexes.

PEPTIDE VACCINE: A vaccine made of synthetic peptides designed to stimulate an immune response by stimulating T cells. Peptide vaccines are HLA restricted since the peptide must bind to a specific HLA complex.

PET SCAN: A positron emission tomography scan is a functional imaging study that identifies highly active cells, such as cancer cells, because they take up large amounts of glucose. PET scans are helpful for finding sites of melanoma throughout the body.

PHASE I TRIAL: A clinical study that evaluates the safety of a drug or device being tested in patients for the first time. Phase I drug studies are based on extensive experimental findings and are approved by the FDA and local IRB in the United States.

PHASE II TRIAL: A clinical study that may extend tests of safety for a drug, and begins to evaluate how effective the new drug works. Phase II studies usually focus on a particular type of cancer.

PHASE III TRIAL: A clinical study that compares a new drug or device to the current standard for treatment. If there is no accepted standard of care, a drug may be compared to no treatment or a placebo treatment.

PIGMENTED SKIN LESIONS: Pigmented lesions refer to skin lesions that contain pigment, generally melanin, and indicates an increase in the number of melanocytes or melanocyte activity. Benign pigmented skin lesions are often called moles or nevi, whereas malignant pigmented skin lesions are melanomas.

PLACEBO: A harmless substance used as a constant in controlled experiments, testing the effectiveness of another substance.

PLAQUE RADIOTHERAPY: A type of treatment for certain forms of ocular melanoma and other eye tumors. The treatment is a form of local radiation therapy and requires a surgical procedure to implant a source of radiation with a protective cap.

POLYMERASE CHAIN REACTION (PCR): A technique in molecular biology that permits the identification of any short sequence of DNA (or RNA). The technique is very sensitive and can find a single gene in one million cells.

PRECLINICAL STUDY: Research using animals or human cells to find out if a drug, procedure, or treatment is likely to be useful. Preclinical studies take place in research laboratories before any testing is done in humans.

PREVENTION TRIAL: A clinical study that evaluates if drugs, other agents, or behavioral changes can reduce the risk of cancer.

PROTEIN KINASES: A family of enzymes that mediate a number of important cell functions, including cell growth and survival. Many protein kinases are abnormal in cancer cells (oncogenes) and blocking protein kinases represents a new strategy for treating cancer.

PUNCH BIOPSY: A type of incisional biopsy in which the doctor removes a portion of a suspicious skin lesion by rotating a cookie cutter-like tool down through the full thickness of the skin to the underlying fat.

RADIATION THERAPY: The treatment of cancer with forms of energy, including X-rays and gamma rays; also called radiotherapy.

RADIONUCLIDE: A small molecule that has an artificial or natural origin and exhibits radioactivity; used for imaging sites of disease and for therapy of some cancers.

RAF KINASE INHIBITOR: A new class of drug that blocks the activity of overactive Raf kinases in melanoma cells. This drug is being tested now in clinical trials.

RANDOMIZED STUDY: A trial in which patients are assigned randomly to receive one or another treatment, possibly including a placebo.

REJECTION: The failure of a recipient's body to accept a transplanted tissue or organ as the result of immunological incompatibility.

RESPONSE RATE: The percentage of patients whose cancer responds after treatment; the response may be complete, partial, or stable.

RETINA: The delicate, multi-layered, light-sensitive membrane lining the inner layer of the eyeball; the retina contains rods and cones, and connects visual images to the brain by the optic nerve.

RETROVIRUS: Viruses that contain RNA as their genetic material, rather than DNA. Retroviruses insert their genetic material into the chromosomes of infected cells, becoming a permanent part of the host cell's genetic material. Retroviruses have been used in gene therapy to deliver new genes into cancer cells.

SATELLITOSIS: Appearance of numerous skin deposits of metastatic melanoma around a primary—or original—melanoma, or at the site of a previously removed melanoma.

SCREENING STUDY: A study or test to detect cancer early in order to minimize its harm.

SEBACEOUS GLAND CARCINOMA: A rare type of skin cancer that arises from the small sebaceous glands located just below the skin. These cancers are often very aggressive.

SEBORRHEIC KERATOSES: A common, benign, raised, waxy-looking lesion resulting from excessive growth of keratinocytes. They can appear on sun-exposed or covered areas, and range in color from tan to dark brown or black.

SENTINEL NODE: The first lymph node or nodes to receive drainage from a melanoma site; the sentinel node is the most likely lymph node to have metastatic disease, if any lymph nodes are involved.

SHAVE BIOPSY: Type of skin biopsy in which the top layers of the skin are "shaved" off with a surgical blade. Shave biopsies are most useful in diagnosing superficial, benign skin diseases that do not require a deep tissue sample. Shave biopsy is not to be done if melanoma is suspected.

SIDE EFFECT: A secondary and usually adverse effect of treatment.

SKIN GRAFT: A procedure where skin from another part of the body is taken to cover a defect in the skin, due to a large surgical excision, for example.

SOMATIC PAIN: Pain caused by the activation of pain receptors in either the surface or deep tissues of the outer body. Somatic pain is usually felt at the site of the nerve endings.

SPF: See *Sun protection factor.*

SPONTANEOUS REGRESSION: The disappearance (complete regression) of cancer without treatment; thought to be related to destruction of cancer cells by the immune system.

SPORADIC MELANOMA: Melanoma that occurs in individuals without a known genetic or inherited predisposition.

SQUAMOUS CELL CARCINOMA: A type of skin cancer arising from squamous cells.

SQUAMOUS CELLS: Flat cells located in the middle layer of the epidermis that produce keratin, an important skin protein providing added protection for the skin.

STROMAL CELLS: A type of cell found in the surrounding tissue of an organ, usually providing structural or other support for the organ cells.

SUBCUTANEOUS: Pertaining to the layer of tissue beneath the skin.

SUBUNGUAL HEMATOMA: A blood collection under the fingernail or toenail.

SUBUNGUAL MELANOMA: This rare form of melanoma occurs under a nail, most often the thumb or big toe, and appears as a brown or black discoloration that is often mistaken for a bruise (hematoma) or infection.

SUNBLOCK: A preparation that prevents sunburn by filtering out the sun's ultraviolet rays, usually offering more protection than a sunscreen.

SUN PROTECTION FACTOR (SPF): The SPF is a number that indicates the time you can stay exposed to the sun without burning. An SPF of 30 or 45 is generally recommended for protection against skin cancer.

SUNSCREEN: A preparation that protects the skin from the ultraviolet rays of the sun.

SUPERFICIAL INGUINAL LYMPH NODE DISSECTION: A surgical procedure involving the removal of lymph nodes in the groin.

SUPERFICIAL SPREADING MELANOMA: The most common type of melanoma, characterized by spreading along the epidermis for months to years before penetrating more deeply into the skin. The melanoma appears as a flat or barely raised lesion, often with irregular borders and variations in color.

SUPPRESSOR T CELL: A T cell that reduces or suppresses the immune response of B cells or of other T cells to an antigen.

SYSTEMIC THERAPY: Any treatment that reaches and affects cancer cells all over the body, such as chemotherapy and immunotherapy.

TARGETED THERAPY: A form of therapy that targets cancer cells while preserving normal cells. It is distinct from chemotherapy, which hits all cells, especially the rapidly dividing cells.

T CELLS: A subset of white blood cells, T cells mature in the thymus, recognize foreign antigens as peptide fragments, and stimulate an immune response which can last for many years.

TEMOZOLAMIDE (TEMODAR): A type of oral chemotherapy used to treat melanoma.

THALIDOMIDE (THALOMID®): A type of oral drug with many anti-cancer properties including stimulation of the immune system and blocking blood vessel growth near cancers. Thalidomide was used as a sedative and anti-nausea drug for pregnant women in the 1950s but caused severe birth defects. Thalidomide, and its derivatives, are being actively tested for many different types of cancer.

THERAPEUTIC TRIAL: A clinical study evaluating the use of drugs, surgical procedures, or other interventions for the treatment of cancer or other diseases.

THYMIDINE KINASE: An enzyme that is important in generating the building blocks of DNA inside cells. A viral form of this enzyme has been used in gene therapy studies by placing the enzyme in cancer cells and adding ganciclovir, a drug that is converted by the enzyme into an agent that blocks DNA formation and cell growth. This approach remains experimental.

TOLL-LIKE RECEPTOR AGONISTS: A new class of molecules which bind to dendritic cells and activate them into mature antigen presenting cells; this may help promote a strong immune response.

TOPICAL CHEMOTHERAPY: Treatment with anti-cancer drugs in a lotion or cream applied to the skin.

TRANSFORMING GROWTH FACTORS: A family of cytokines that may inhibit or block normal immune responses.

TRANSPUPILLARY THERMOTHERAPY: A method of delivering heat to the back of the eye using an infrared laser. This results in an area of localized heating (hyperthermia), which may be helpful for treating certain eye diseases, including melanoma.

TRICYCLIC ANTIDEPRESSANT: A class of antidepressants that treat depression and may have some benefit in alleviating some forms of cancer related pain.

TUMOR: An abnormal mass of tissue resulting from excessive cell division.

They may either be benign or malignant, but perform no useful body function. See also *cancer*, *lesion*, and *nodule*.

TUMOR-INFILTRATING LYMPHOCYTES: Lymphocytes, typically T cells, that have left the bloodstream and migrated into a tumor.

TUMOR NECROSIS FACTOR ALPHA: A type of cytokine that causes tumor death in animals and is being tested as an experimental immunotherapy, especially in isolated limb perfusion.

TUMOR REGRESSION: A decrease in the size of a tumor or cancer.

TUMOR SUPPRESSOR GENE: Genes in the body that can suppress or block the development of cancer. These may be missing in some cancer cells.

TYROSINASE: A melanoma antigen.

TYROSINASE-RELATED PROTEIN-1: A melanoma antigen.

TYROSINASE-RELATED PROTEIN-2: A melanoma antigen.

ULCERATION: A condition in which the epidermis covering a portion of a primary melanoma is not intact. Ulceration is determined by microscopic evaluation of the tissue by a pathologist and confers a worse prognosis than for melanomas of the same size without ulceration.

ULTRASOUND: An imaging technique that uses ultrasonic waves for diagnostic or therapeutic purposes, specifically to visualize an internal body structure, monitor a developing fetus, or generate localized deep heat to body tissues.

ULTRAVIOLET (UV) A RAYS: Long-wavelength ultraviolet rays given off by the sun, tanning beds, and sunlamps. UVA rays enter the skin more deeply than UVB rays, cause premature aging of the skin, and are believed to cause skin cancer.

ULTRAVIOLET (UV) B RAYS: Medium-wavelength burning rays of the sun that are the primary cause of sunburn. They are considered the main cause of basal and squamous cell carcinoma, as well as a significant cause of melanoma.

ULTRAVIOLET (UV) RADIATION: Also called ultraviolet light, UV radiation is a part of sunlight that is invisible to the human eye. Some wavelengths of UV radiation filter through the earth's atmosphere and enter the body through the skin and eyes. At higher doses, UV radiation can burn the skin and cause melanoma and other types of skin cancer.

VACCINE THERAPY: A treatment strategy whereby parts of a cancer cell are used to stimulate an immune response against the cancer. Although numerous types of vaccines have been developed for melanoma, the approach remains experimental.

VASCULAR ENDOTHELIAL GROWTH FACTOR (VEGF): A substance made by cells that stimulates new blood vessel formation, an essential requirement for continued growth of many cancers.

VIDEOANGIOGRAPHY: An imaging tool that takes pictures after injecting a dye into the small blood vessels in the eye. This technique is especially useful for distinguishing a melanoma from a hemorrhage.

VINBLASTINE (VELBAN): A type of chemotherapy used to treat melanoma.

VINCRISTINE (ONCOVIN): A type of chemotherapy used to treat melanoma.

VIRAL VACCINE: Vaccine in which a virus can be used to carry genes that help to activate an immune response.

VIRUS: A small organism that reproduces itself inside a living cell and is composed of DNA or RNA surrounded by a protein coat. Many viruses cause disease.

VISCERAL PAIN: Pain from the internal organs. Visceral pain is caused by activation of pain receptors resulting from infiltration, compression, extension, or stretching of the internal organs.

VITILIGO: An autoimmune skin disorder of unknown cause involving loss of pigmentation in patches of otherwise normal skin.

WHITE BLOOD CELL (WBC): A type of blood cell that helps the immune system fight infection and disease. White blood cells include lymphocytes, granulocytes, macrophages, and others.

WHOLE CELL VACCINES: Vaccines made from whole tumor cells that have been changed in the laboratory. They can be from a patient (autologous) or derived from other cancer patients (allogeneic).

WIDE LOCAL EXCISION: The standard surgical procedure for early-stage primary melanoma, in which the melanoma—including the biopsy site—and a margin of normal skin are removed. The goal is complete removal of the melanoma.

XERODERMA PIGMENTOSUM: A rare, inherited condition associated with an inability to repair DNA damage caused by ultraviolet radiation. Patients must avoid sun exposure and are at extremely high risk for skin cancer and melanoma.

Acknowledgments

I HAVE SEVERAL people to thank for their contributions to my career and support for this book. My decision to study medicine was influenced by my grandfather, Dr. Albert D. Coyne, who was also an early role model for how to treat patients with compassion and dignity. I am indebted to Dr. Paul LoGerfo, a former colleague who urged me to write this book and helped me understand how important it was to get this information to patients and their families. I was fortunate to have superb surgeons during my training, including Dr. Jack Pickleman, Dr. James Menzoian, Dr. Robert Beazley, Dr. Erwin Hirsch, Dr. Michael T. Watkins, and Dr. Harvey Pass. My early scientific career was inspired by Dr. Judy Kantor, who taught me how to conduct basic laboratory research. My professional life was significantly influenced by interacting with a few giants in academic medicine, such as Dr. Jeffrey Schlom, Dr. Glenn Steele, Dr. Barry Bloom, Dr. Matthew Scharff, and Dr. Karen Antman. I have also been fortunate to work with numerous colleagues whose fierce commitment to finding new treatments for patients with cancer constantly encourages my own work. These individuals who merit thanks include Dr. Mary L. (Nora) Disis, Dr. Robert S. DiPaola, Dr. Franco Marincola, Dr. Jedd Wolchok, and Dr. H. Kim Lyerly. I would like to thank my colleagues in New York City who help take care of my patients, including Dr. Charles Hesdorffer, Dr. Steve Isaacson, Dr. Desiree Ratner, Dr. David Lee, and Dr. Joe Divito. The Melanoma Center exists because of the vision of Dr. David Bickers. I also thank Dr. Eric Rose for his continued support. I would like to acknowledge the many post-doctoral fellows, technicians, students, and data managers who have contributed to building our program. I want to specially thank Margaret Robbins for the author's photograph on the book jacket. I first met Margaret in 2001 when she became my patient. I remember her telling me that of all the difficulties she had to face because of her advanced disease, the worst was that she had lost her interest in photography. Four years after I treated her, she is doing well and, as you can tell from the photo, back to her favorite hobby. Finally, I am indebted to my agent and editor, Robin Dellabough of Lark Productions, for her enthusiasm and hard work on this project; and to Erin Moore at Gotham Books for her critical review of the text and helpful suggestions.

Index

Note: Page numbers in **bold** indicate chapters.
Page numbers in *italics* indicate photograph and illustrations.

About the Author

Dr. Howard L. Kaufman is founder and Co-Director of the Columbia University Melanoma Center, attending physician at the New York-Presbyterian Hospital Columbia University Medical Center, chief of surgical oncology, and associate professor of surgery at Columbia University College of Physicians and Surgeons. He has conducted numerous clinical research trials on vaccines for cancer, lectures widely on cancer treatment, and has published more than one hundred articles in the field of tumor immunology and immunotherapy. He lives in New York City.